THE
ANATOMY
OF THE
HORSE

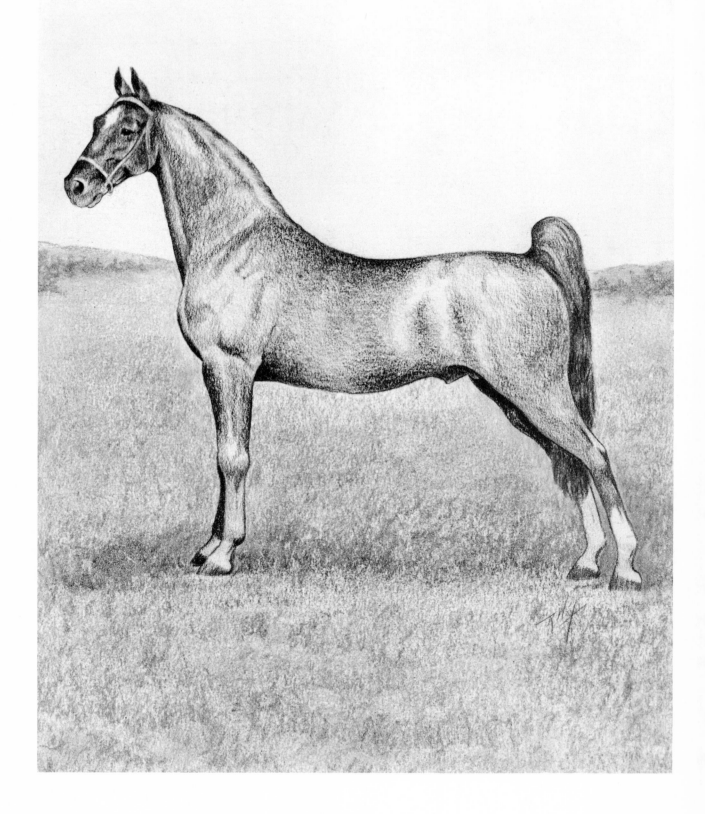

THE
ANATOMY
OF THE
HORSE

A PICTORIAL APPROACH

Robert F. Way, V.M.D., M.S.

Formerly Assistant Professor of Anatomy,
School of Veterinary Medicine
University of Pennsylvania

Donald G. Lee, V.M.D.

Professor of Anatomy and Associate Dean,
School of Veterinary Medicine
University of Pennsylvania

J. B. LIPPINCOTT COMPANY
PHILADELPHIA AND TORONTO

ISBN-0-397-50142-1

Library of Congress Catalog Card Number 64-7778

Printed in The United States of America

7   6

PREFACE

This work incorporates in one volume a series of plates portraying the basic anatomic features of the horse and is designed to permit those interested to become familiar with these features without reading extensive descriptive texts. It is the conviction of the authors that descriptions of anatomic structures are of little value if a specimen is not available for observation. Without material for dissection, one is forced to form mental images of the described structures, and these are seldom correct.

Anatomy is a visual subject. One must either observe a specimen, appropriately dissected, or depend upon accurately reproduced illustrations to form correct mental images. Obviously, it is much easier and less time consuming to utilize illustrations, but a good understanding of the anatomy of any animal can only be gained in this way if the illustrations are accompanied by legends directing the observers' attention to important structures.

While many treatises have been published on the anatomy of the horse, no atlas is available at the present time with legends in the English language. The major aim of the authors is, therefore, to provide a volume which will acquaint the artist, the horse lover, and the veterinary student with the anatomic features of the horse with a minimum of effort.

ROBERT F. WAY
DONALD G. LEE

INTRODUCTION

The modern horse is an herbivorous quadruped specialized, as a result of natural selection and selective breeding, for the attainment of speed. Its digestive system is adapted for the efficient handling of food of plant origin and its body and appendages streamlined for agility, speed, and endurance.

The evolutionary history of the horse is well known and provides the clues needed to understand and interpret its anatomic peculiarities. Practically the earliest recognizable equine animal is Eohippus of the Lower Eocene period. This animal was but 12 inches high and had a short head and neck. Its forefoot possessed four weight-bearing toes with a rudimentary medial splint bone indicating a five-toed ancestry. The hind foot had three functional toes and a lateral splint bone. Since it is customary to designate the most medial digit as number one and to number the other digits in order outward, it follows that in Eohippus the first digit of the forefoot was rudimentary, while the first digit of the hind foot had completely disappeared and the fifth or lateral digit had become rudimentary. In tracing the further evolution of the horse through Mesohippus of Lower Oligocene time, Merychippus in the Miocene, to Pliohippus of Pleocene time, we find a gradual reduction in the number of digits. Pliohippus was the first one-toed horse having on both fore and hind feet a functional third digit and rudimentary second and fourth digits represented by the medial and lateral splint bones. The same condition exists in the genus Equus, which includes a number of Pliocene and Pleistocene fossil forms, as well as in the living horses of today. In the modern horse we have, therefore, a highly evolved animal of large size totally dependent on the functional integrity of but one functional digit upon which it prances in the manner of a ballet dancer.

As a result of the reduction in the number of digits there has occurred a number of other anatomical modifications. These involve a reduction in the number of muscles in the antebrachial or forearm region of the thoracic limb and in the tibial region of the rear limb. Many muscles corresponding to those of the hand and foot of primates have completely disappeared, others have become rudimentary, while others have evolved into strong, primarily ligamentous structures to provide the extra support required.

A knowledge of the anatomy of the horse is essential for one to understand its physiologic processes, to develop proper husbandry methods, and to diagnose and treat the disease conditions to which it is prone.

All of the illustrations in this atlas are reproduced from original drawings made by one of the authors (R.F.W.), the majority from his own dissections of actual specimens. The legends for the drawings were prepared by the collaboration of both authors. The terminology utilized was kept as simple as possible by anglicizing the Latin terms of conventional anatomic nomenclature.

CONTENTS

SECTION ONE
The Anatomy of the Head.................................... 1

SECTION TWO
The Muscles of the Neck and the Trunk................. 17

SECTION THREE
The Body Cavities and Viscera............................ 43

SECTION FOUR
The Genitalia...................................... 53

SECTION FIVE
The Appendicular Skeleton and the Bones of the
Front Limb.................................... 63

SECTION SIX
The Pectoral Region and the Front Limb.............. 79

SECTION SEVEN
The Bones of the Hind Limb................................139

SECTION EIGHT
The Hind Limb..161

INDEX...207

SECTION ONE

The Anatomy of the Head

PLATE 1

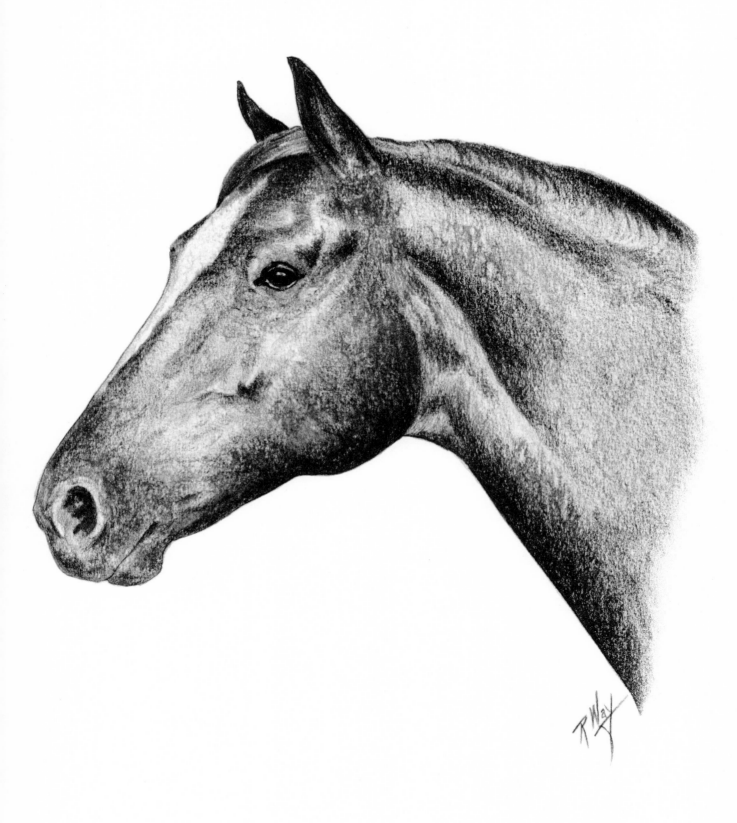

(Plate 1)   3

PLATE 2

The superficial muscles of the head

1. Orbicularis oris
2. Mentalis
3. Depressor labii inferioris
4. Buccinator
5. Zygomaticus
6. Dilatator naris lateralis
7. Levator labii superioris proprius
8. Levator nasolabialis
9. Fronto-scutularis
10. Parotido-auricularis
11. Masseter
12. Sternocephalicus
13. Brachiocephalicus
14. The jugular vein

Note: It should be pointed out for those who are familiar with human anatomic terminology that the sternocephalicus (12) and the brachiocephalicus (13) correspond to the sternocleidomastoideus and the clavicular head of the deltoideus of the human.

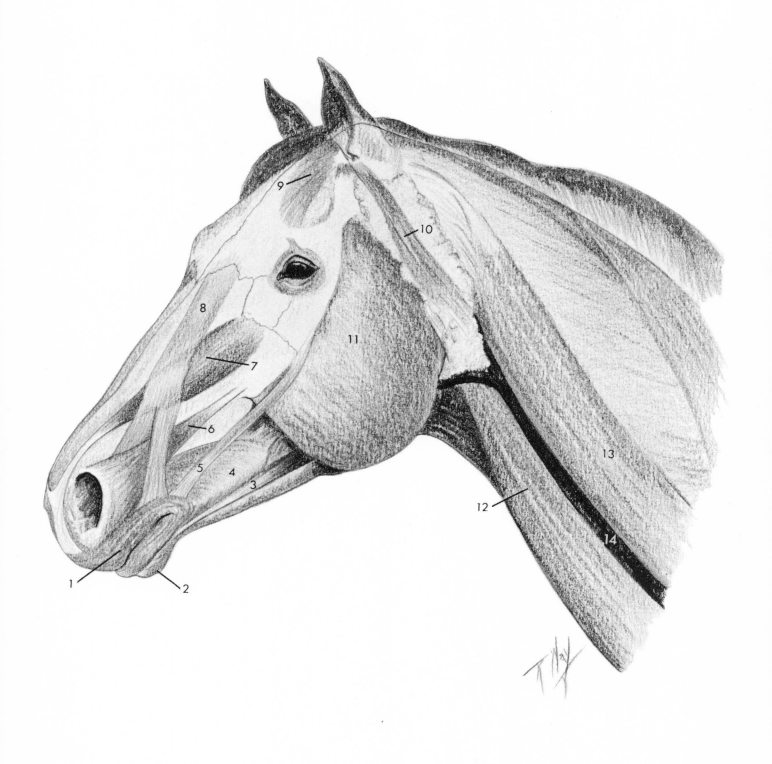

(Plate 2)   5

PLATE 3

The bones of the head

1. Premaxilla or incisive bone, which contains the alveoli for the upper incisor teeth
2. Maxilla, which contains the alveoli for the premolar and the molar teeth
3. Infra-orbital foramen
4. Nasal bone
5. Frontal bone
6. Supra-orbital process of the frontal bone
7. Parietal bone
8. Occipital bone
9. Squamous portion of the temporal bone
10. External auditory meatus in the petrous portion of the temporal bone
11. Coronoid process of the mandible
12. Mandible, which bears the alveoli for all the teeth of the lower jaw
13. Zygomatic bone
14. Lacrimal bone
15. Atlas or 1st cervical vertebra
16. Axis or 2nd cervical vertebra

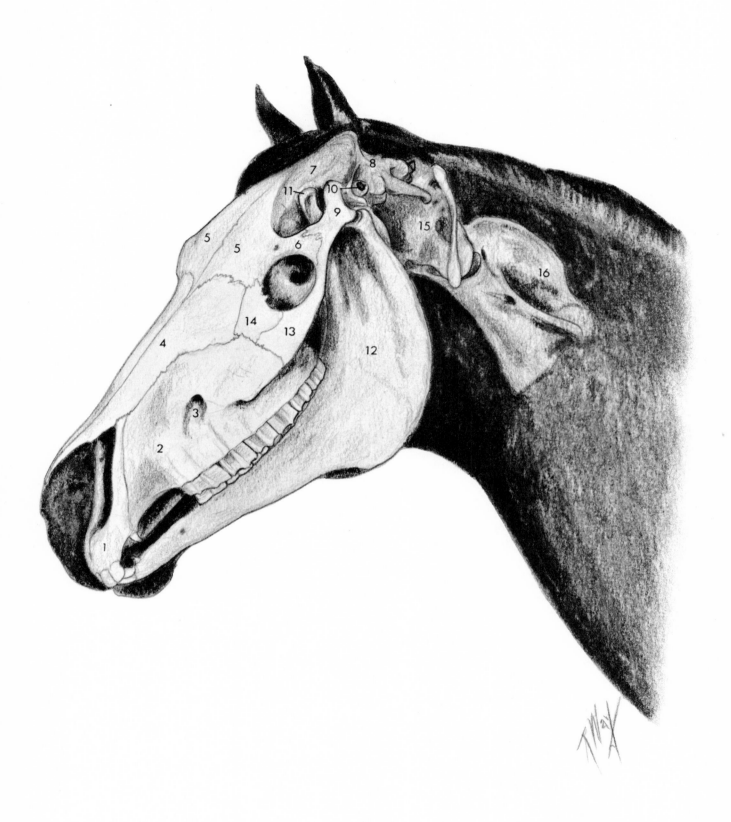

(Plate 3)   7

PLATE 4

The cavities of the skull

1. Nasal cavity
2. Frontal sinus. The outer plate of the frontal bone has been partially removed.
3. Cranial cavity, exposed by removal of a portion of the parietal bone
4. Orbital cavity
5. Maxillary sinus, exposed by removal of a large portion of the outer plate of the maxilla

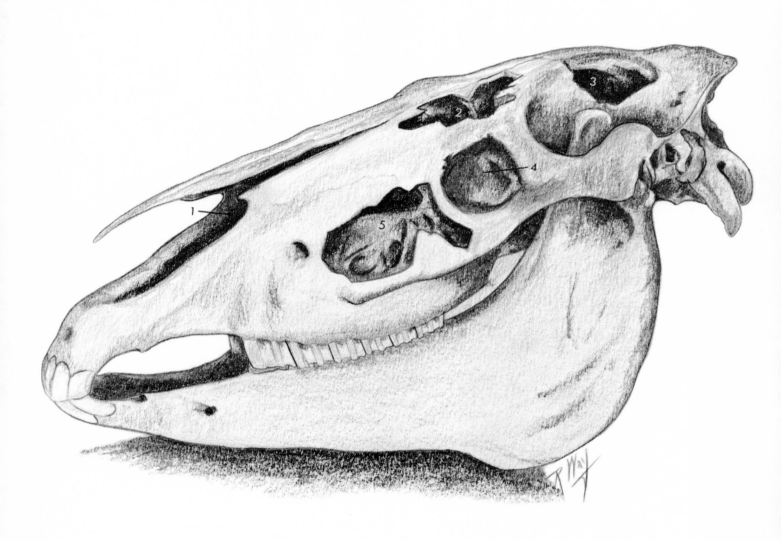

(Plate 4)   9

PLATE 5

The superficial vessels and nerves of the head

1. Jugular vein
2. The 3rd cervical nerve
3. The 2nd cervical nerve
4. Cutaneous nerve of the neck
5. Caudal auricular nerve
6. Branches of the 1st cervical nerve
7. Caudal auricular vein
8. Masseteric vein and artery
9. External maxillary vein
10. Facial nerve, which provides motor innervation to the muscles of expression
11. Auriculo-palpebral branch of the facial nerve
12. Superficial temporal vein
13. Transverse facial vein and artery
14. Transverse facial nerve
15. Superior buccal branch of the facial nerve
16. Inferior buccal branches of the facial nerve
17. Facial vein and artery
18. Inferior labial artery
19. Superior labial vein and artery
20. Lateral nasal vein and artery
21. Angular artery and vein

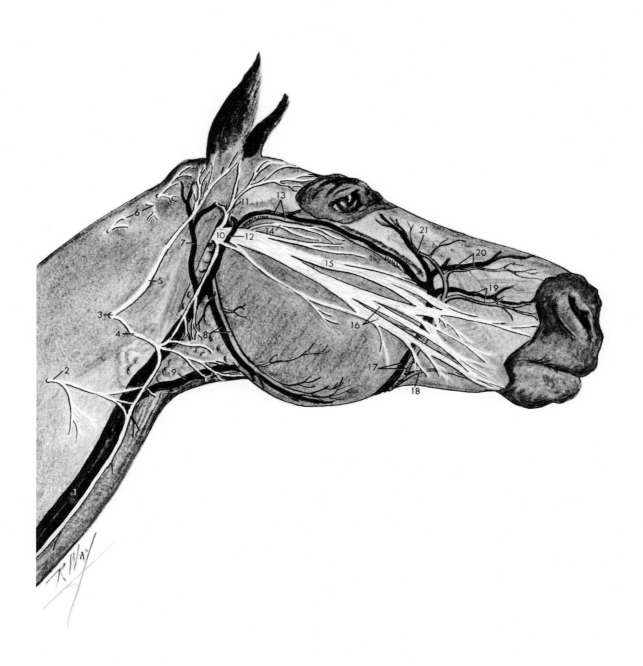

(Plate 5)   11

PLATE 6

The superficial structures on the ventral aspect of the head

1. Cranial end of the brachiocephalicus muscle
2. Cranial end of the sternocephalicus muscle
3. Cranial end of the sternohyoideus and the omo-hyoideus muscles

4. Ventral end of the parotid salivary gland
5. Duct of the parotid salivary gland. This conveys the secretion of the gland to the oral opening of the duct opposite the 3rd upper cheek tooth.
6. External maxillary artery and vein. The pulse may be taken most conveniently where the artery crosses the ventral edge of the mandible.
7. Mandibular lymph node
8. Mylohyoideus muscle
9. Ventral border of the mandibular ramus
10. Body of the mandible

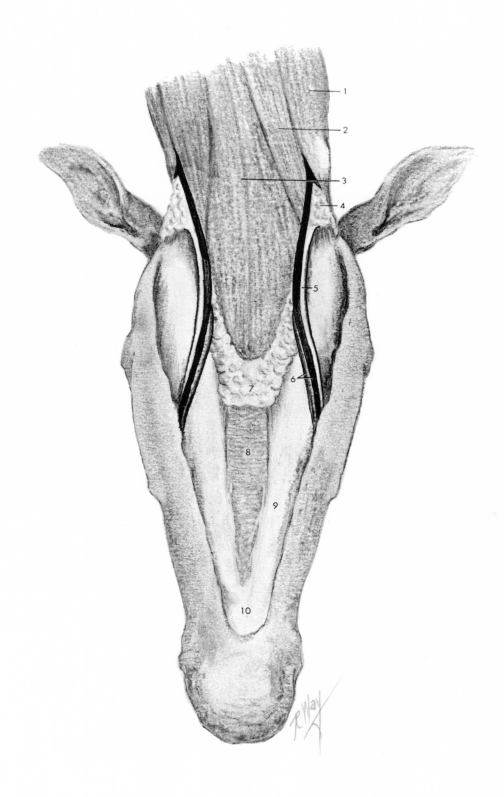

(Plate 6) 13

PLATE 7

The structures visible in a longitudinal median section of the head

1. Funicular portion of the ligamentum nuchae
2. Rectus capitis dorsalis muscle
3. Dorsal arch of the atlas
4. Ventral arch of the atlas
5. Rectus capitis ventralis muscle
6. Esophagus
7. Lamina of the cricoid cartilage of the larynx
8. Lumen of the trachea
9. Arch of the cricoid cartilage
10. Lumen of the larynx
11. Vocal fold
12. Lateral ventricle of the larynx
13. Epiglottis
14. Body of the thyroid cartilage of the larynx
15. Cranial end of the sternohyoideus muscle
16. Hyo-epiglotticus muscle
17. Soft palate
18. Longitudinal lingual muscle
19. Hyoid bone
20. Mylohyoideus muscle
21. Geniohyoideus muscle
22. Genioglossus muscle
23. Body of the mandible
24. Mentalis muscle
25. Incisor teeth
26. Rostral tip of the tongue
27. Oral cavity
28. Body of the premaxilla
29. Hard palate
30. Inferior nasal meatus through which the stomach tube is passed
31. Ventral turbinate
32. Middle nasal meatus
33. Dorsal turbinate
34. Dorsal nasal meatus
35. Ethmoturbinates
36. Lumen of the pharynx
37. Fold which covers the pharyngeal orifice of the auditory (or Eustachian) tube
38. Lumen of the gutteral pouch, a ventral diverticulum of the auditory tube peculiar to the Equidae
39. Lumen of the sphenopalatine sinus
40. Lumen of the frontal sinus
41. Medial surface of the left cerebral hemisphere
42. Cerebellum
43. Medulla oblongata

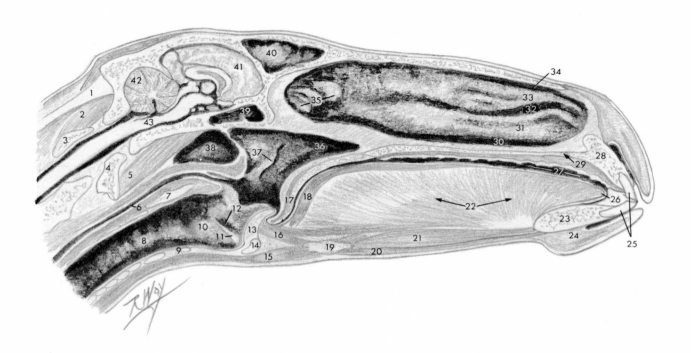

(Plate 7)   15

SECTION TWO

The Muscles of the Neck and the Trunk

PLATE 8

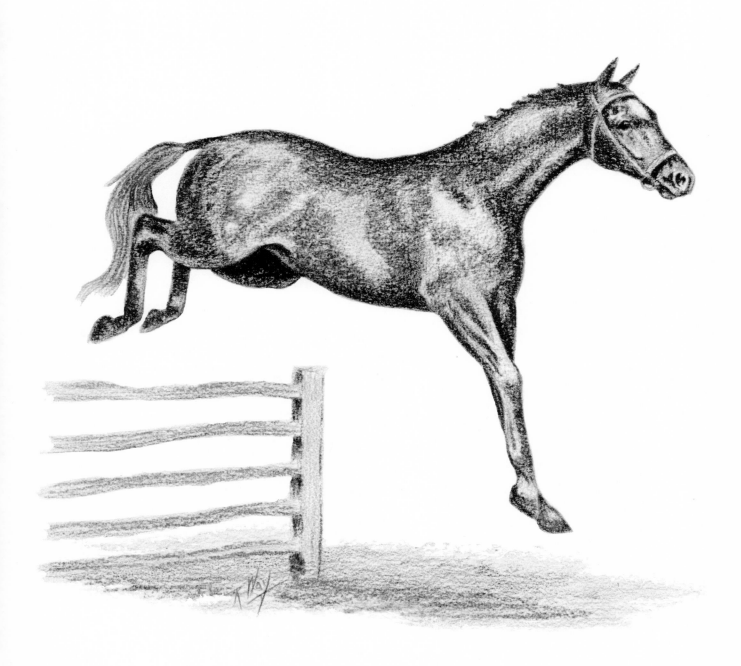

(Plate 8)   19

PLATE 9

The superficial muscles of the horse in action. All muscles illustrated here are labeled on Plates 11 and 36.

Note that the front limbs are in the extended position and that at the time of impact with the ground the entire weight of the animal will be absorbed by the left front limb. This places tremendous strain on the supporting structures of the limb.

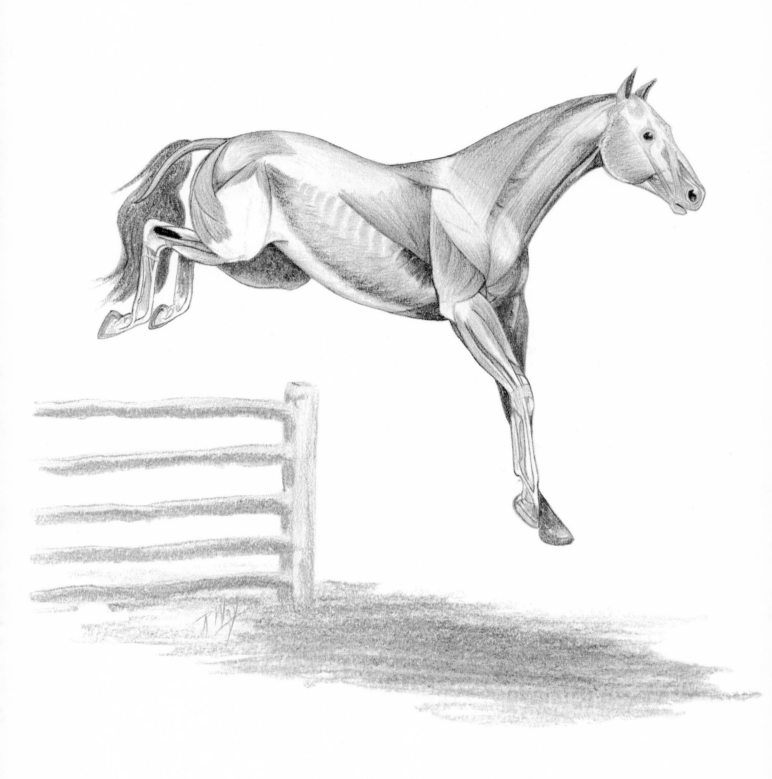

(Plate 9)   21

PLATE 10

The skeleton of the horse in action, illustrating both the axial and the appendicular portions

The skeleton of the limbs is fully illustrated in Plates 28, 29, 63 and 65

1. Atlas or 1st cervical vertebra
2. Axis or 2nd cervical vertebra, constructed to permit rotatory movements of the head as well as flexion and extension
3. Cervical vertebrae, nos. 3 to 7
4. Thoracic vertebrae. There are 18 thoracic vertebrae, all of which may be distinguished by their high spines. The spines of the 3rd and 4th form the highest point of the withers.
5. Lumbar vertebrae, which may be distinguished by their long flat transverse processes. There are typically 6 lumbar vertebrae.
6. Sacrum, formed by fusion of 5 sacral vertebrae
7. Coccygeal vertebrae, which vary in number from 15 to 21
8. Sternum, which consists of 6 to 8 bony segments, the sternebrae, connected to each other by cartilage. The first 8 pairs of ribs articulate with the sternum. Note that the sternum forms the floor of the thoracic cavity.
9. Ribs, of which there are 18 pairs. These form the bony support for the lateral walls of the thoracic cavity.

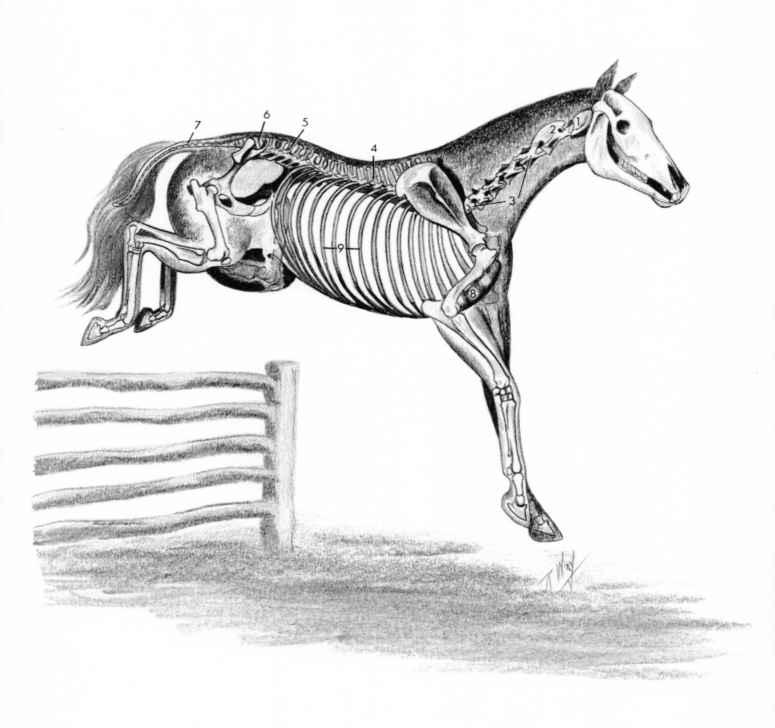

(Plate 10) 23

PLATE 11

A superficial dissection of the muscles of the neck, the shoulder, the trunk and the pelvic regions

1. Brachiocephalicus. Note that this muscle extends over the shoulder to insert on the humerus.
2. Splenius
3. Rhomboideus cervicalis
4. Trapezius cervicalis
5. Serratus ventralis cervicis
6. Cutaneous colli
7. Trapezius thoracalis
8. Deltoideus
9. Long head of the triceps brachii
10. Latissimus dorsi
11. Serratus ventralis thoracis
12. Caudal deep pectoral muscle
13. External abdominal oblique muscle
14. Tensor fasciae latae
15. Gluteus medius
16. Gluteus superficialis
17. Biceps femoris
18. Semitendinosus

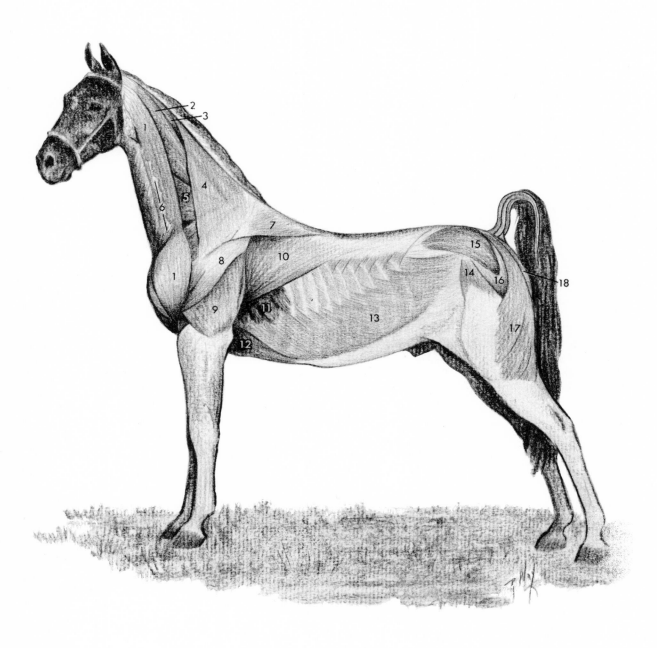

(Plate 11) 25

PLATE 12

This plate differs from the preceding in that some of the superficial muscles have been removed, namely, trapezius cervicalis, trapezius thoracalis, deltoideus, and latissimus dorsi. This exposes the next layer of muscles in the cervical and the thoracic areas.

1. Brachiocephalicus
2. Splenius
3. Rhomboideus cervicalis
4. Rhomboideus thoracalis
5. Serratus ventralis cervicis
6. Cranial deep pectoral muscle
7. Supraspinatus
8. Infraspinatus
9. Long head of the triceps brachii
10. Serratus ventralis thoracis
11. Serratus dorsalis cranialis
12. Serratus dorsalis caudalis
13. External intercostals

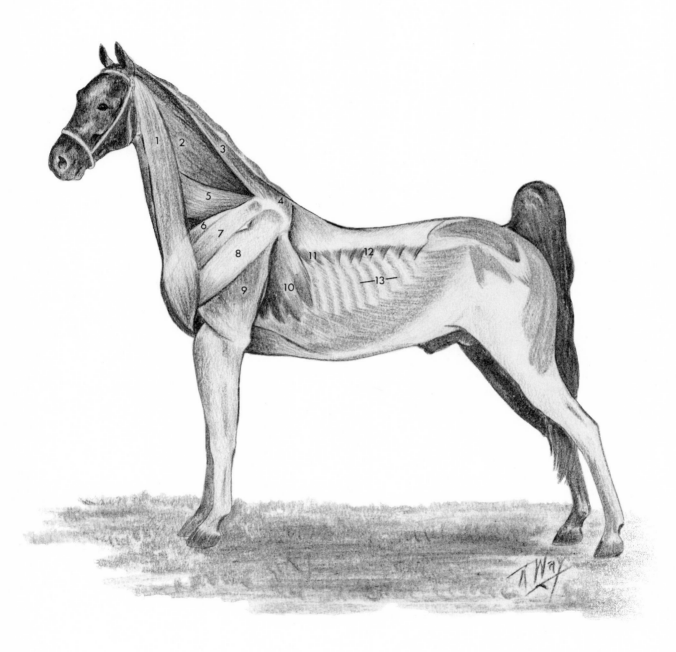

(Plate 12) 27

PLATE 13

This plate is intended to illustrate chiefly the muscles which lie medial or deep to the shoulder and the arm, which have been removed.

1. Rhomboideus thoracalis
2. Rhomboideus cervicalis
3. Splenius
4. Serratus ventralis cervicis
5. Serratus ventralis thoracis
6. Cranial superficial pectoral muscle
7. Cranial deep pectoral muscle
8. Caudal deep pectoral muscle
9. Caudal superficial pectoral muscle
10. Cranial portion of the external abdominal oblique muscle

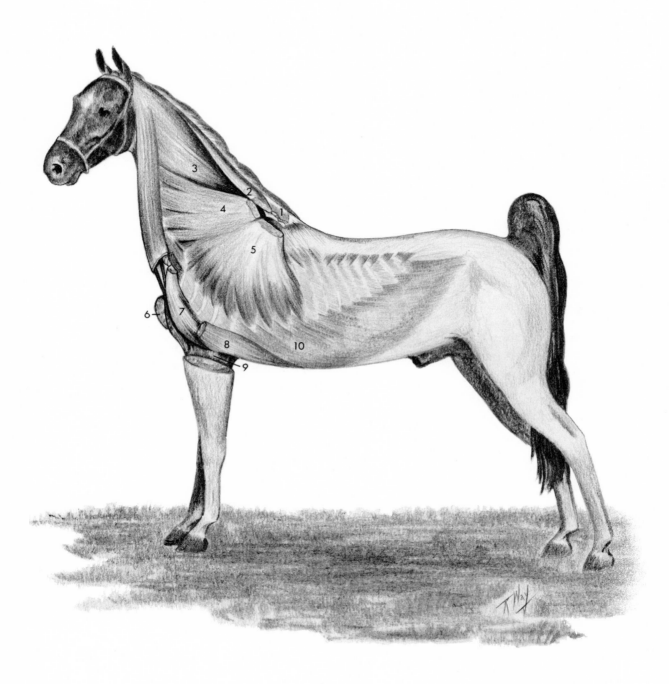

(Plate 13)   29

PLATE 14

A slightly deeper dissection of the muscles of the cervical region than is illustrated in the preceding plate. Here the rhomboideus, the serratus ventralis and the pectoral muscles have been removed.

1. The wide, flat splenius muscle
2. Longissimus cervicis muscle
3. Scalenus muscle, illustrating the dorsal and the ventral portions
4. Trachea
5. Cut end of the brachiocephalicus muscle
6. Caudal end of the sternocephalicus muscle
7. Lateral aspect of the sternum
8. Transversus costarum (or rectus thoracis) muscle
9. Cranial end of the rectus abdominis muscle
10. Wide, flat external abdominal oblique muscle
11. Aponeurosis of insertion of (10)
12. Oval hole in the aponeurosis of the external abdominal oblique, which forms the external inguinal ring
13. Longissimus dorsi muscle
14. Iliocostalis muscle

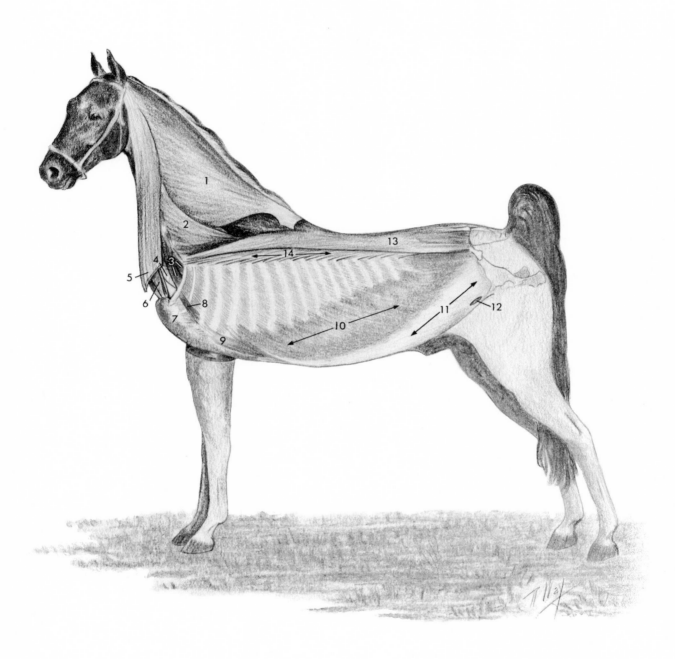

(Plate 14)   31

PLATE 15

This plate illustrates some of the deeper muscles of the neck, the epaxial muscles and the deeper muscles of the abdominal wall. The left shoulder and arm have been removed as well as the following superficial muscles: cutaneous colli, brachiocephalicus, splenius, serratus ventralis, serratus dorsalis, trapezius, rhomboideus, pectorals, and the obliquus abdominis externis.

1. Stump of the transected cutaneous colli
2. Sternocephalicus muscle
3. Trachea
4. The two portions of the scalenus muscle
5. Rectus capitis ventralis major muscle
6. Longissimus atlantis muscle
7. Longissimus capitis muscle
8. Longissimus cervicis muscle
9. Longissimus dorsi muscle
10. The wide, flat semispinalis capitis muscle
11. Funicular portion of the ligamentum nuchae
12. Spinalis et semispinalis muscle
13. Iliocostalis muscle
14. Transversus costarum (or rectus thoracis) muscle
15. Rectus abdominis muscle
16. Obliquus abdominis internus muscle. Note that its ventral aponeurosis (16′) extends over the ventral abdominal wall superficial to the rectus abdominis.

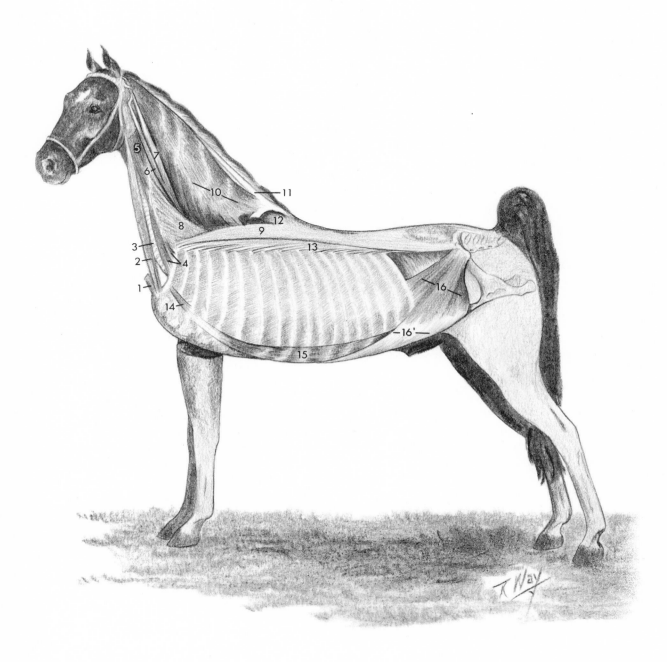

(Plate 15)   33

PLATE 16

This plate is similar to the preceding one except that the sternocephalicus, the semispinalis capitis and the obliquus abdominis internus muscles have been removed to illustrate more deeply lying muscles.

1. Sterno-thyro-hyoideus muscle
2. Trachea
3. Rectus capitus ventralis major muscle
4. Obliquus capitis caudalis muscle
5. Obliquus capitis cranialis muscle
6. Multifidis cervicis muscle
7. Intertransversarii muscles
8. Lamellar portion of the ligamentum nuchae
9. Funicular portion of the ligamentum nuchae
10. Spinalis and semispinalis dorsi and cervicis muscles
11. Multifidis dorsi muscle
12. Longissimus dorsi muscle
13. Iliocostalis muscle
14. Transversus costarum (or rectus thoracis) muscle
15. Rectus abdominis muscle
16. Transversus abdominis muscle. Note that its aponeurosis (16') lies deep to the rectus abdominis muscle and its tendon of insertion.

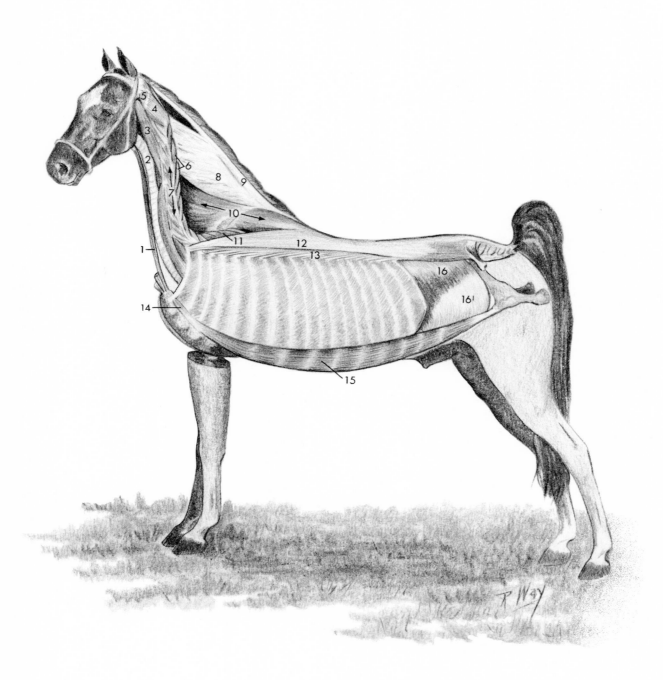

(Plate 16)   35

PLATE 17

This plate differs from the preceding one in that the longissimus dorsi, the spinalis and semispinalis dorsi and cervicis, the intercostals and the rectus abdominis muscles have been removed. This exposes the deepest epaxial muscles, the ribs, the costal cartilages, the lungs and the diaphragm.

1. The ligamentum nuchae, which is composed of 2 strong elastic cords (the funicular portion) extending from the spines of the thoracic vertebrae forward to the head and 2 sheetlike lamellae (constituting the lamellar portion) lying side by side (1'), which extend from the thoracic spines downward and forward to attach to the spines of the 2nd and to the 6th cervical vertebrae. This elastic ligament permits the horse to support the head and the neck without muscular exertion.
2. Supraspinous ligament
3. Multifidis dorsi muscle — a series of bundles arising from the transverse processes of the thoracic vertebrae and extending obliquely forward and upward to insert on the spines of the thoracic vertebrae.
4. Multifidis lumborum — a series of bundles arising from the articular processes of the lumbar vertebrae and extending forward and upward to the lumbar vertebral spines.
5. Levatores costarum — a series of small muscles arising from the transverse processes of the thoracic vertebrae and inserting on the cranial borders of the ribs.
6. The ribs. The horse usually has 18 pairs of ribs; 8 of these articulate with the sternum and are called sternal ribs, and 10 do not articulate with the sternum and are called asternal ribs.
7. Sternum
8. The costal cartilages, one for each rib. They attach the sternal ribs to the sternum. Those of the asternal ribs collectively form the costal arch.
9. Left lung
10. Diaphragm
11. The transversus abdominis muscle, the deepest muscle of the abdominal wall. Note that its aponeurosis lies deep to the rectus abdominis, which has been removed except for a small portion of its caudal end.

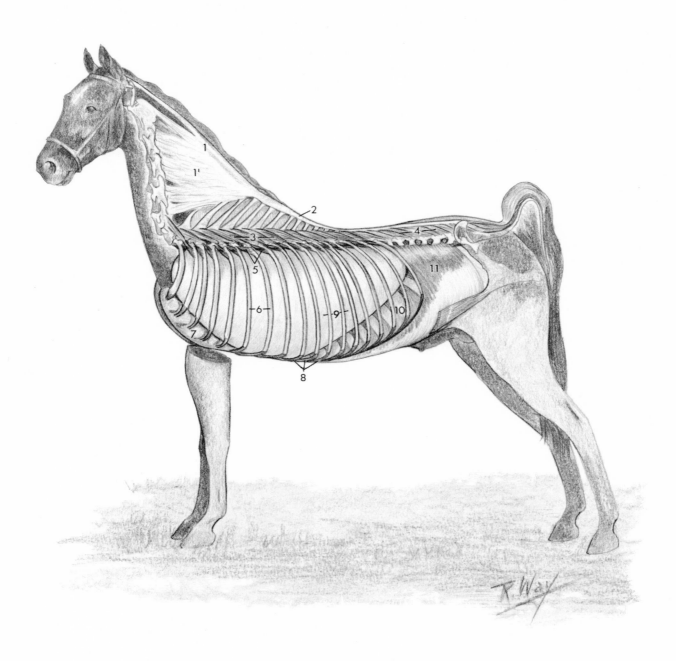

(Plate 17)   37

PLATE 18

The external or subcutaneous inguinal ring. The left leg has been removed from the os coxae or hip bone and the femoral lamina of the aponeurosis of the external oblique abdominal muscle has been removed with the leg.

1. The high insertion of the muscular fibers of the external oblique abdominal muscle onto the tuber coxae
2. The lateral cutaneous nerves from lumbar nerves 1 and 2 emerging between the muscular fibers of the external oblique abdominal muscle
3. Lateral cutaneous nerve of the thigh (lumbar 3) emerging through the aponeurosis of the external oblique abdominal muscle in company with the caudal branch of the circumflex iliac artery
4. Severed cranial portion of the iliacus muscle lying beneath the wing of the ilium
5. The large femoral nerve, which has been cut in removing the limb, running ventrally behind the iliacus and lateral to the whitish tendinous fibers of insertion of the psoas minor muscle
6. Cut ends of the external iliac artery and vein emerging under the tendon of insertion of the psoas minor muscle
7. Origin of the rectus femoris muscle from two depressions on the ilium
8. Origin of the small capsularis muscle
9. The deep acetabulum in which the head of the femur articulates
10. Slit or opening in the aponeurosis of the external oblique abdominal muscle which is the external or subcutaneous inguinal ring
11. The very strong prepubic tendon
12. Accessory ligament of the hip joint
13. Stump of the obturator nerve
14. Obturator artery

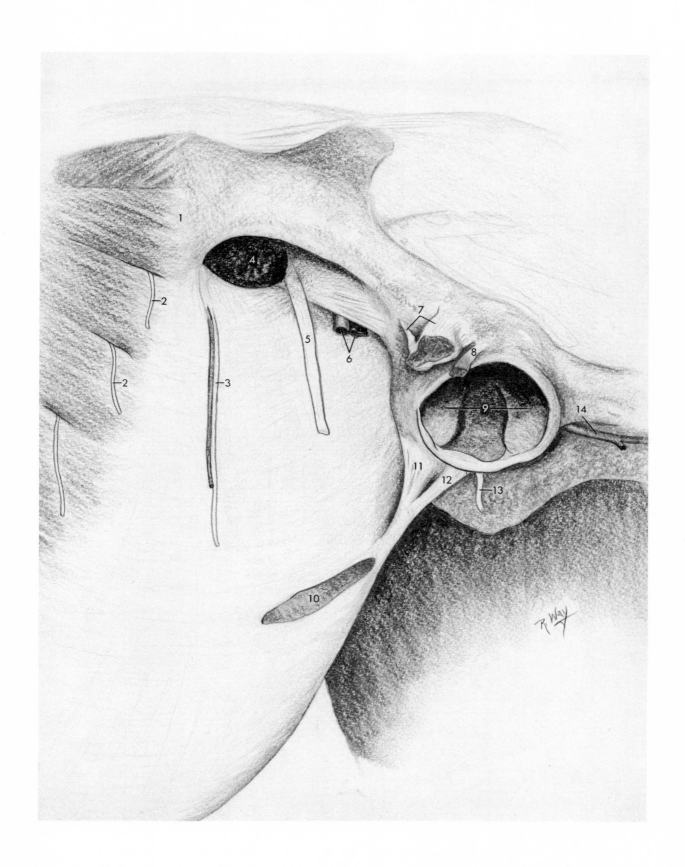

(Plate 18)   39

PLATE 19

The internal oblique abdominal muscle. The left rear leg has been removed and the aponeurosis of the external oblique abdominal muscle incised, allowing the caudal part to hang ventrally.

1. The origin of the internal oblique abdominal muscle from the tuber coxae
2. The insertion of the internal oblique abdominal muscle dorsally onto the last rib and the costal arch by muscular fibers and, ventrally, by means of a broad aponeurosis which joins the aponeurosis of the external oblique abdominal muscle
3. The direction of the muscular fibers of the internal oblique. Note that the cranial fibers run downward and forward and the caudal fibers run downward and backward. The muscle is more or less fan shaped.
4. The lateral cutaneous nerve of the thigh emerging under the iliacus muscle in company with the caudal branch of the circumflex iliac artery
5. The muscular branch of the external spermatic nerve (lumbar 3) descending over the peritoneum and bifurcating to supply the internal oblique and the external cremaster muscles. The inguinal branch of the same nerve has been cut.
6. The peritoneum and its tubular evagination, the tunica vaginalis, which has been cut
7. The external cremaster muscle has been dissected away from the tunica vaginalis communis to show the evagination to better advantage.
8. The short, cut stump of the prepubic artery and its bifurcation into the caudal deep epigastric artery and the external pudendal artery which can be seen passing through the external inguinal ring

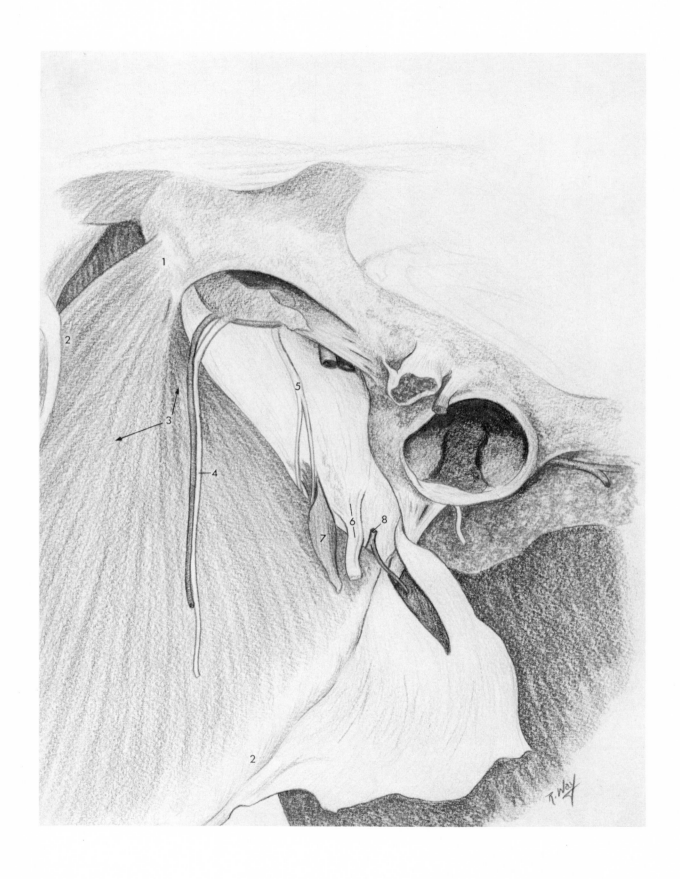

(Plate 19)   41

SECTION THREE

The Body Cavities and Viscera

PLATE 20

The vessels and the nerves of the right side of the thorax. The ribs and the right lung have been removed (after Ellenberger, Leisering's Atlas, 2nd Edition, Leipzig, 1899).

1. The heart covered by the pericardium
2. Caudal vena cava
3. Azygos vein. Note the segmental intercostal veins which drain into it.
4. Cranial vena cava
5. Costocervical vein
6. Vertebral vein
7. Internal thoracic vein
8. External thoracic vein
9. Stump of the axillary vein from the right front limb
10. Cephalic vein
11. Jugular vein
12. External maxillary vein
13. Internal maxillary vein
14. Common carotid artery
15. Bicarotid trunk
16. Vertebral artery
17. The point of bifurcation of the omocervical artery into ascending and descending branches
18. Costocervical artery
19. External thoracic artery
20. Internal thoracic artery
21. Stump of the axillary artery
22. Brachiocephalic artery
23. Thoracic aorta
24. The great thoracic lymph duct
25. The sympathetic trunk
26. A ramus communicans connecting the sympathetic trunk to a spinal nerve
27. Intercostal artery, vein and nerve
28. Diaphragm
29. Phrenic nerve
30. Ventral esophageal nerve running ventral to the esophagus
31. Dorsal esophageal nerve
32. The roots of the brachial plexus, here shown reflected upward
33. The cervical portion of the sympathetic trunk
34. Recurrent laryngeal nerve
35. Vagus nerve
36. Spinal accessory nerve shown descending over the splenius muscle and terminating on the trapezius muscle

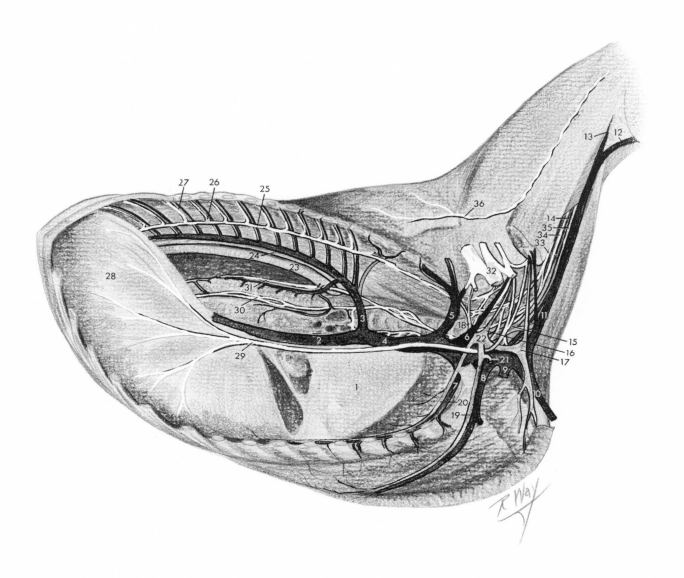

(Plate 20)   45

PLATE 21

Vessels and nerves of the left side of the thorax. The ribs have been removed and the left lung incised and reflected downward to expose the left pulmonary artery (after Ellenberger).

1. The heart with pericardial sac removed
2. Descending branch of the left coronary artery
3. Circumflex branch of the left coronary artery
4. Pulmonary artery
5. Thoracic aorta
6. Phrenic artery
7. Common brachiocephalic artery
8. Left subclavian artery
9. Costocervical artery
10. Deep cervical artery
11. Vertebral artery
12. The bicarotid trunk, which gives rise to right and left common carotids (12′)
13. Omocervical artery
14. Stump of the left axillary artery
15. Stump of the external thoracic artery
16. Internal thoracic artery
17. Stump of the left axillary vein
18. Stump of the left jugular vein
19. The great lymphatic duct which empties into the precaval vein at (19′)
20. The recurrent laryngeal nerve lying ventral to the left common carotid artery; (20′) is its point of origin from the vagus nerve.
21. Combined vagus nerve and cervical portion of the sympathetic trunk
22. The nervus transversarius, which represents the combined gray rami communicantes connecting the sympathetic trunk to the cervical spinal nerves Nos. 2-7
23. Cardio-sympathetic and cardio-vagal nerve fibers
24. Pulmonary nerves
25. Dorsal and ventral esophageal branches of the vagus nerve
26. The sympathetic trunk
27. The greater splanchnic nerve
28. Esophagus
29. Severed branches of the left bronchus
30. Trachea
31. Thyroid gland

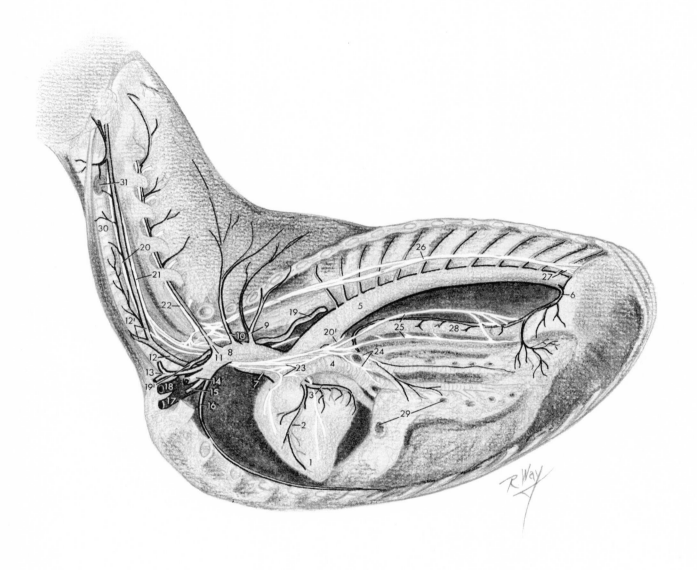

(Plate 21)   47

PLATE 22

Lateral view of thoracic and abdominal cavities. The ribs and the intercostal muscles have been removed to show the thoracic viscera; the abdominal wall has been removed to show the abdominal viscera.

Figure 1. Left lateral view.

1. Scapula
2. Humerus
3. Proximal end of the ulna
4. Proximal end of the radius
5. The heart

6. Cardiac notch of the lung
7. Parietal surface of the lung
8. Basal border of the lung
9. Muscular rim of the diaphragm
10. Costal arch
11. Left ventral portion of the great colon
12. Coils of the small intestine
13. Coils of the small or descending colon
14. Os coxae

Figure 2. Right lateral view.

(1) through (10) as for Figure 1
11. Right ventral portion of the great colon
12. Body of the caecum
13. Base of the caecum
14. Pelvic flexure of the great colon
15. Os coxae

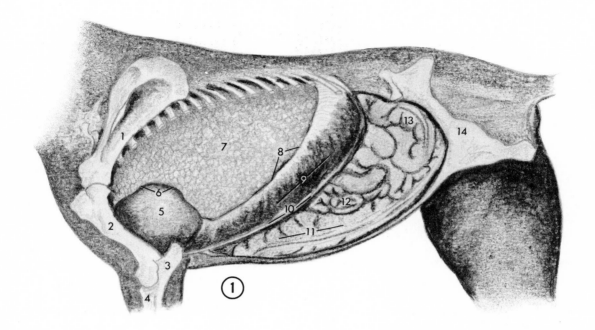

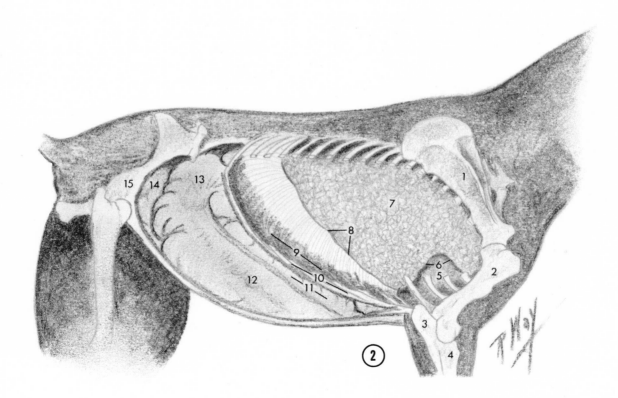

(Plate 22)   49

PLATE 23

The pelvic inlet of a stallion. The animal has been completely transected in the midlumbar region and the observer is looking caudally into the pelvic cavity.

1. Three major structures in the pelvic cavity; the rectum dorsally, genital fold in the center, and the bladder on the pelvic floor
2. The mesorectum attached to the dorsal surface of the rectum
3. Free cranial edge of the genital fold extending to the vaginal rings, where it is continued ventrally as the mesorchium enclosing the spermatic cord
4. Vaginal rings
5. Middle ligament of the bladder extending forward toward the umbilicus
6. The large pubic bones with a median eminence (male)
7. The caudal deep epigastric artery and 2 collateral veins running cranially beneath the peritoneum
8. The aorta with the caudal vena cava on its right surface
9. The deep circumflex iliac arteries with their 2 collateral veins running outward beneath the peritoneum
10. The cut ends of the 2 ureters which are descending into the pelvic cavity toward the urinary bladder
11. The internal iliac lymph glands are barely visible at the terminal bifurcation of the aorta
12. The cut lumbar vertebra, with the small paired psoas minor muscles situated ventromedially against the body and the psoas major muscles, much larger, situated under the transverse processes and over the psoas minor muscles. Above the transverse processes note the small multifidus dorsi muscles situated along the sides of the spinous processes and the sacrospinalis muscles occupying the remainder of the space.
13. Ventrally, note the cut muscular substance of the 2 rectus abdominis muscles running between the aponeurosis of the transversus abdominal muscle internally and the combined aponeuroses of the 2 oblique abdominal muscles externally.

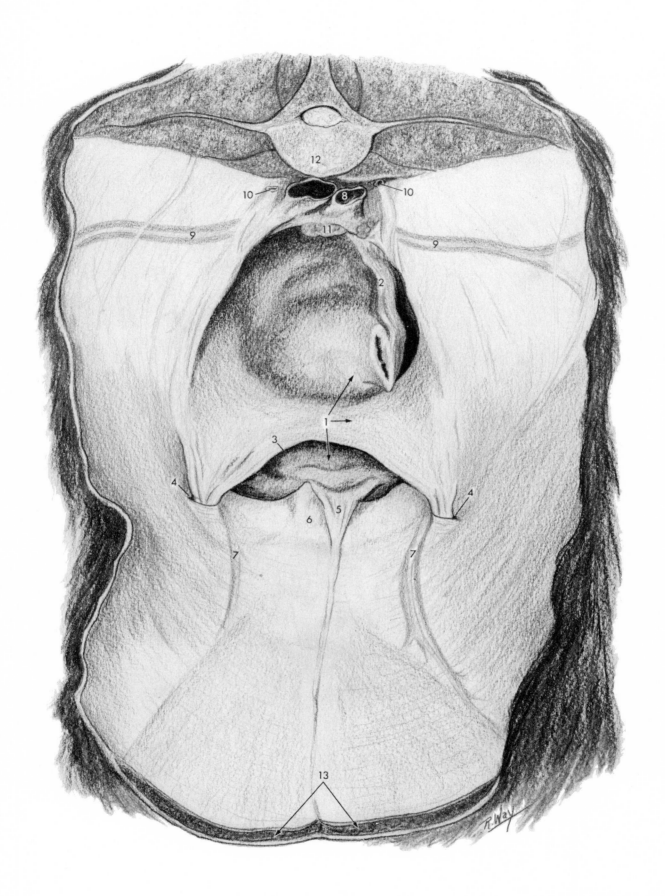

(Plate 23)   51

SECTION FOUR

The Genitalia

PLATE 24

Diagrammatic representation of the arrangement of the male genital organs

1. Right testicle, lying in the right scrotal sac
2. Right spermatic cord
3. Right ductus deferens
4. Genital fold
5. Urinary bladder, which lies ventral to the genital fold
6. Left spermatic cord entering the abdominal ring of the inguinal canal
7. Left ductus deferens
8. Right seminal vesicle
9. Prostate gland
10. Pelvic portion of the urethra
11. Bulbo-urethral gland
12. Penis
13. Rectum

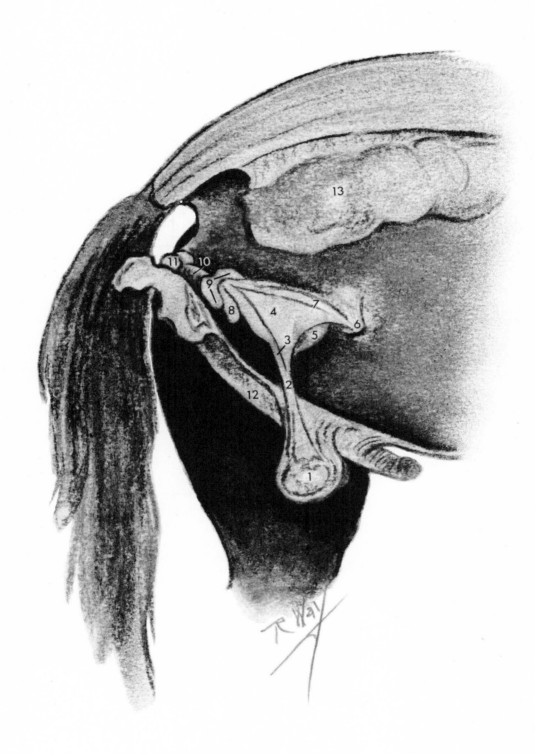

(Plate 24)   55

PLATE 25

The external genitalia of a yearling colt. The animal has been placed on its back and the skin of the scrotum, the prepubic region and medial surfaces of the thighs has been reflected. The dartos of the scrotum and the scrotal fascia have been removed.

1. Preputial orifice
2. Skin of the prepuce
3. Right and left (3') superficial inguinal lymph nodes situated on either side of the penis, each lying lateral to a caudal superficial epigastric artery
4. Left subcutaneous inguinal ring

5. Tunica vaginalis communis covering the 2 small testes
6. Right and left external cremaster muscles inserting on the tunica vaginalis communis
7. Retractor penis muscle which extends along the ventral surface of the penis
8. Fibers of the bulbocavernosus muscle covering the corpus cavernosum urethrae of the penis
9. Left and right (9') ischiocavernosus muscles which ensheath the two crura of the penis from their attachment at the ischial arch to the body of the penis. Large segments of the semimembranosus muscle have been removed in order to show these completely.
10. External anal sphincter
11. Anus
12. Gracilis muscle
13. Semimembranosus muscle

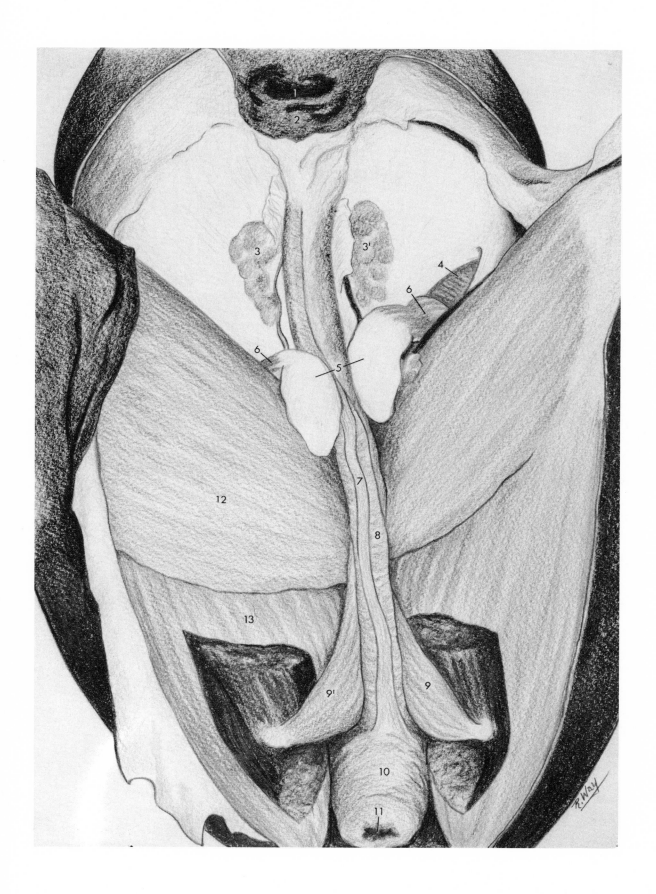

(Plate 25)   57

PLATE 26

Inguinal structures of a yearling colt. The animal is placed on its back and the skin of the scrotum, the prepubic region and the medial surfaces of the thighs has been reflected. The suspensory ligament of the penis has been severed, permitting it to be reflected caudad.

1. Superficial inguinal lymph node
2. External spermatic nerve
3. Caudal superficial epigastric artery
4. Subcutaneous inguinal ring
5. External pudendal artery, which divides into 2 terminal branches, (3) and (6)
6. Cranial dorsal artery of the penis
7. Tunica vaginalis communis covering the under-developed left testicle
8. Stump of the external pudendal vein
9. Gracilis muscle
10. Semimembranosus muscle
11. Left dorsal nerve of the penis
12. Penis

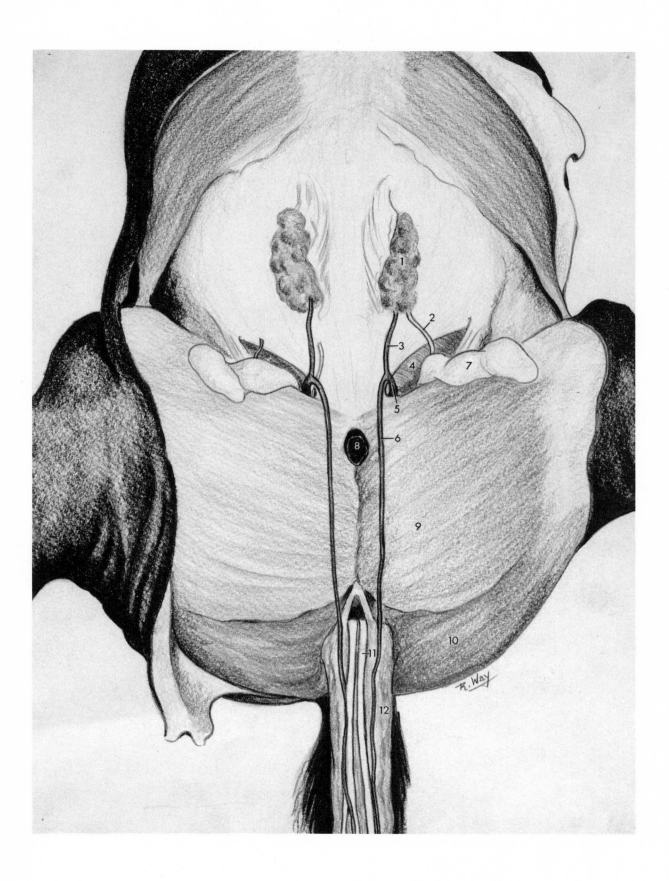

(Plate 26)   59

PLATE 27

Semidiagrammatic illustration of the urogenital system and the pelvic viscera of the mare

1. Left kidney
2. Left ureter. Note that this continues caudad to terminate by opening into the neck of the urinary bladder (12).
3. The utero-ovarian artery, which divides into ovarian and cranial uterine branches
4. Middle uterine artery
5. The broad ligament
6. Umbilical artery
7. Left ovary
8. Coiled left oviduct
9. Round ligament of the uterus
10. Left uterine cornua or horn
11. Body of the uterus
12. Urinary bladder
13. Urethra
14. Vagina
15. Rectum
16. Rectococcygeus muscle
17. Sphincter ani externus
18. Anus
19. Constrictor vestibuli muscle
20. Constrictor vulvae muscle
21. Vulvar cleft

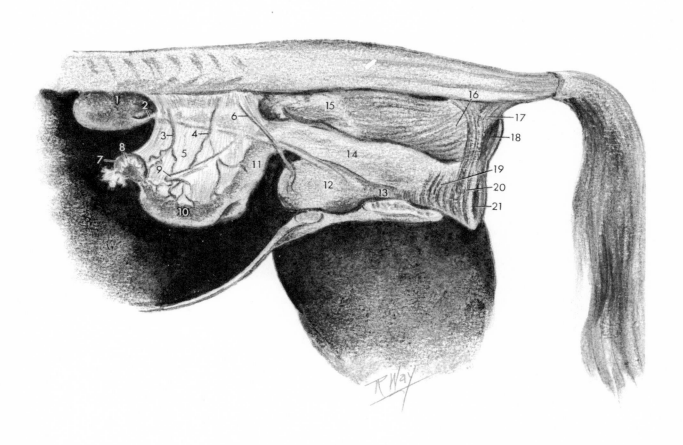

(Plate 27) 61

SECTION FIVE

The Appendicular Skeleton
and the Bones of the
Front Limb

PLATE 28

The appendicular skeleton as seen from the lateral aspect

1. Scapula—the bone of the shoulder
2. Humerus—the bone of the arm or brachium
3. Ulna
4. Radius, which together with the ulna makes up the skeleton of the forearm or antebrachium. In the horse the radius is much the larger of these two bones, while the size of the ulna is reduced as compared to other mammals.
5. Bones of the carpus. In the human these are the bones which make up the wrist, but the horseman refers to this region as the knee of the horse. Anatomically this is incorrect usage.
6. Lateral or 4th metacarpal or splint bone. There is a similar medial or 2nd metacarpal splint bone which is not visible.
7. Large or 3rd metacarpal

8. Lateral proximal sesamoid. The medial proximal sesamoid is not illustrated.
9. First phalanx or long pastern
10. Second phalanx or short pastern
11. Third phalanx or coffin bone
12. Ilium
13. Pubis
14. Ischium. The ilium, the ischium and the pubis fuse together to form the os coxae. This joins with its fellow of the opposite side ventrally at the symphysis pelvis to form the pelvic girdle.
15. Femur, or thigh bone
16. Patella, or knee cap
17. Fibula
18. Tibia. The tibia and fibula together form the skeleton of the leg or crus. In the horse the fibula is greatly reduced in size as compared to that of primates.
19. Bones of the tarsus
20. Lateral or 4th metatarsal, or splint bone. The medial or 2nd metatarsal is illustrated on the right hind limb.
21. Third metatarsal, or cannon bone

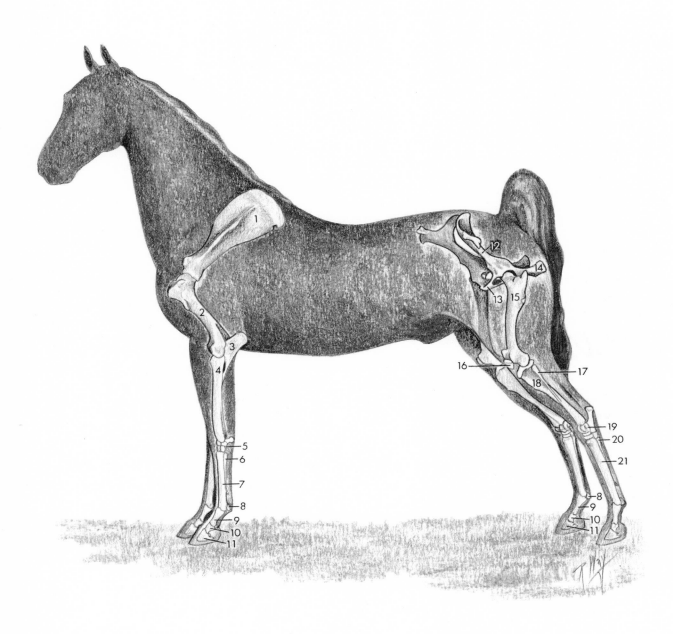

(Plate 28)   65

PLATE 29

The bones of the front limb as seen from the medial aspect

1. The scapula
2. The humerus
3. The ulna, which in the horse is reduced in size as compared with other mammals and is fused to the radius. This prevents movements of supination and fixes the limb in a pronated position.
4. The radius
5. The carpus. This is composed of 7 or 8 in-dividual bones arranged in 2 rows. The horse-man refers to this region as the "knee" but, on a comparative anatomic basis, it is not the knee but the wrist.
6. & 7. The small metacarpal bones, often termed "splint" bones. The one on the medial aspect is the 2nd metacarpal and the one on the lateral aspect is the 4th metacarpal. Both are rudimen-tary and represent nonfunctional vestiges of the 2nd and the 4th digits.
8. The large or 3rd metacarpal bone. In the horse the 3rd digit is the functional digit.
9. The proximal sesamoid bones, 2 in number.
10. The first phalanx or long pastern
11. The 2nd phalanx or short pastern
12. The 3rd phalanx or coffin bone
13. The distal sesamoid or navicular bone

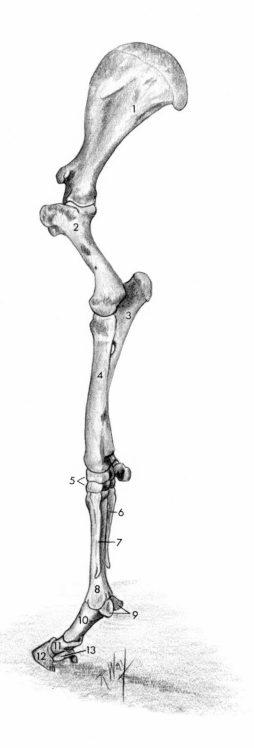

(Plate 29)   67

PLATE 30

Areas of muscular attachment on the scapula. In all figures corresponding areas are numbered identically.

Figure 1. The lateral surface.
Figure 2. The medial surface.
Figure 3. The distal end.

1. Scapular cartilage. In Figure 2 the black area represents the area of insertion of the rhomboideus muscle.
2. The prominence is the scapular tuberosity and the cross-hatched area is the origin of the biceps brachii muscle.
3. Coracoid process, from which the coracobrachialis muscle originates

4. Area of origin of the teres major muscle
5. Area of origin of the long head of the triceps brachii muscle
6. Areas of origin of the teres minor muscle
7. Spine of the scapula
8. Area of insertion of the trapezius cervicalis and thoracalis muscles
9. Supraspinous fossa. Cross-hatching indicates the area of origin of the supraspinatus muscle.
10. Infraspinous fossa. Cross-hatching indicates the area of origin of the infraspinatus muscle.
11. Area of origin of the deltoideus muscle
12. Area of attachment of the serratus ventralis muscle
13. Subscapular fossa. Cross-hatching indicates area of origin of the subscapularis muscle.
14. Area of origin of the capsularis muscle
15. Glenoid cavity, for articulation with the head of humerus

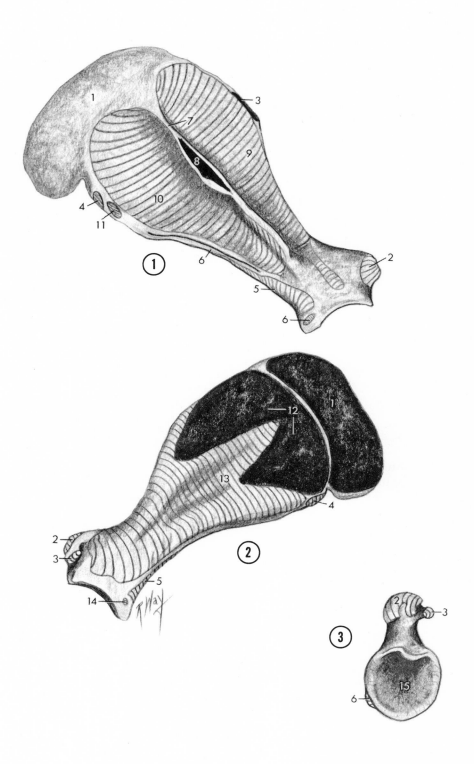

(Plate 30)   69

PLATE 31

Areas of muscular attachment on the humerus. In all figures corresponding figures are numbered identically.

    Figure 1. Distal end.
    Figure 2. Lateral aspect.
    Figure 3. Proximal end.
    Figure 4. Cranial aspect.
    Figure 5. Medial aspect.
    Figure 6. Caudal aspect.

1. Area of origin of the ulnaris lateralis muscle
2. Olecranon fossa
3. Area of origin of the humeral heads of the superficial and the deep digital flexor muscles
4. Area of origin of the flexor carpi ulnaris muscle
5. Area of origin of the flexor carpi radialis muscle
6. Medial condyle and (7) lateral condyle, which articulate with the proximal ends of the radius and the ulna
8. Areas of insertion of the supraspinatus muscle
9. Areas of insertion of the infraspinatus muscle
10. Area of insertion of the teres minor muscle
11. Area of origin of the lateral head of the triceps brachii muscle
12. Area of origin of the brachialis muscle
13. Deltoid tuberosity and site of insertion of the deltoideus muscle
14. Site of origin of the extensor carpi radialis muscle
15. Area of origin of the anconeus muscle
16. Areas of origin of the common digital extensor muscle
17. Area of insertion of the caudal deep pectoral muscle
18. Area of insertion of the subscapularis muscle
19. Head of the humerus, which articulates with the glenoid cavity of the scapula to form the shoulder joint
20. Teres tuberosity—the site of insertion of the conjoined tendons of the latissimus dorsi and teres major muscles
21. Area of insertion of the coracobrachialis muscle
22. Elongated line of attachment of the brachiocephalicus muscle
23. Site of origin of the medial head of the triceps brachii muscle
24. Site of insertion of the capsularis muscle

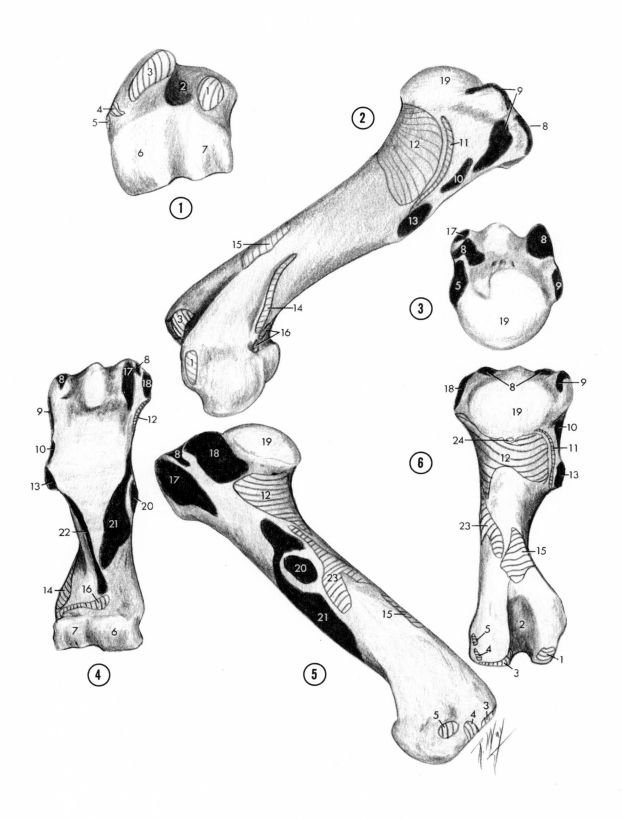

(Plate 31)   71

PLATE 32

Areas of muscular attachment on the radius and the ulna. In all figures corresponding areas are numbered identically.

Figure 1. Medial aspect of the proximal end of the radius and the ulna.

Figure 2. Lateral aspect.

Figure 3. Caudal aspect.

Figure 4. Cranial aspect — proximal portions.

1. Areas of insertion of the triceps brachii muscle
2. Area of origin of the ulnar head of the flexor carpi ulnaris muscle
3. Area of origin of the ulnar head of the deep digital flexor muscle
4. Articular surfaces of the ulna and the radius which articulate with the condyles of the humerus
5. The area where the biceps brachii muscle inserts
6. Insertion area of the brachialis muscle
7. Area of insertion of the tensor fascia antebrachii muscle
8. Area of insertion of the anconeus muscle
9. One of the radial origins of the common digital extensor muscle
10. Radial origin of the lateral digital extensor muscle
11. Ulnar origin of the lateral digital extensor muscle
12. Second radial origin of the common digital extensor muscle. This continues downward on the shaft of the ulna.
13. Area of origin of the extensor carpi obliquus muscle
14. Origin of radial head of the deep digital flexor muscle
15. The radial origin of the superior check ligament (the radial head of the superficial digital flexor muscle)

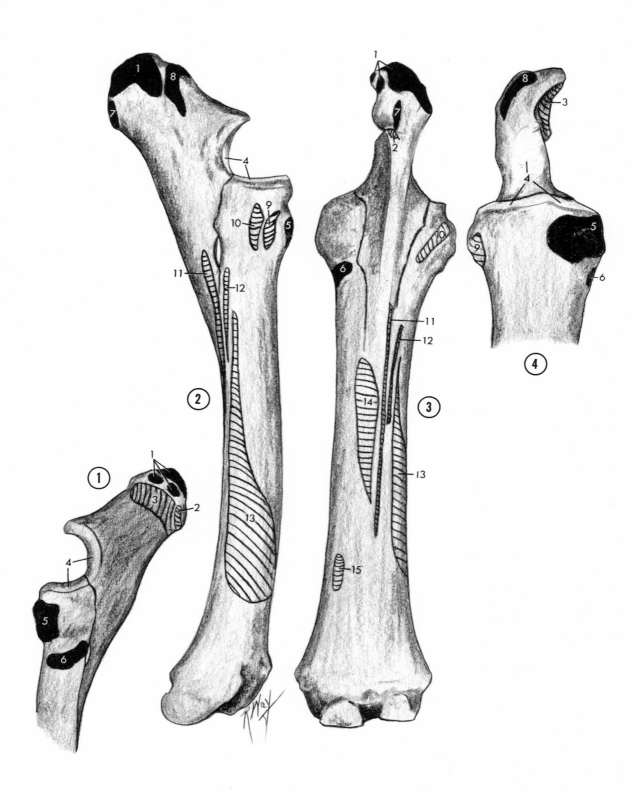

(Plate 32)   73

PLATE 33

The bones of the carpus. The carpus consists of 7 or 8 small bones arranged in 2 rows. There are always 4 bones in the proximal row and 3 or 4 bones in the distal row.

Figure 1. Cranial view.
Figure 2. Lateral view.
Figure 3. Medial view.
Figure 4. Caudal view.

In all figures the corresponding bones are numbered as follows:

1. Radial carpal bone
2. Intermediate carpal bone
3. Ulnar carpal bone
4. Accessory carpal bone
5. Second carpal bone
6. Third carpal bone
7. Fourth carpal bone
8. First carpal bone (this is sometimes missing)

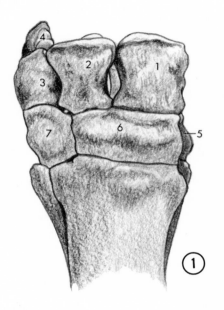

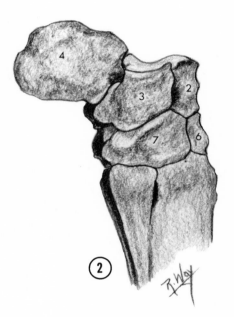

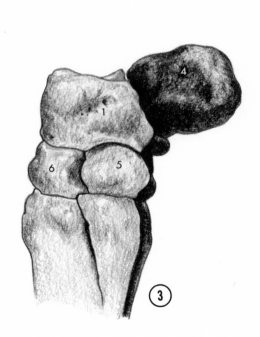

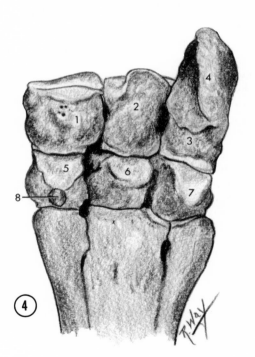

(Plate 33)   75

PLATE 34

Carpus, metacarpus, and digit, showing areas of muscular attachment.

Figure 1. Lateral aspect.
Figure 2. Cranial aspect
Figure 3. Medial aspect.
Figure 4. Volar or caudal aspect.

In all figures the corresponding bones are numbered as follows:

1. Distal end of the radius
2. Radial carpal bone
3. Intermediate carpal bone
4. Ulnar carpal bone
5. Accessory carpal bone
6. First carpal bone
7. Second carpal bone
8. Third carpal bone
9. Fourth carpal bone
10. Third metacarpal bone
11. Second metacarpal bone—often termed the lateral "splint" bone
12. Fourth metacarpal bone or medial "splint" bone
13. Medial and lateral proximal sesamoid bones
14. First phalanx or long pastern
15. Second phalanx or short pastern
16. Third phalanx or coffin bone
17. Distal sesamoid or navicular bone

Muscle attachments
a. The areas of insertion of the ulnaris lateralis muscle
b. Insertion area of the flexor carpi ulnaris muscle
c. Insertion area of the extensor carpi radialis muscle
d. The areas of origin of the interosseous muscle or suspensory ligament of the fetlock
e. Point of insertion of the extensor carpi obliquus muscle
f. Insertion area of the flexor carpi radialis
g. Insertion areas of the suspensory ligament
h. The point of insertion of the lateral digital extensor
i. Insertion areas of the superficial digital flexor
j. Insertion area of the common digital extensor
k. Insertion area of the deep digital flexor

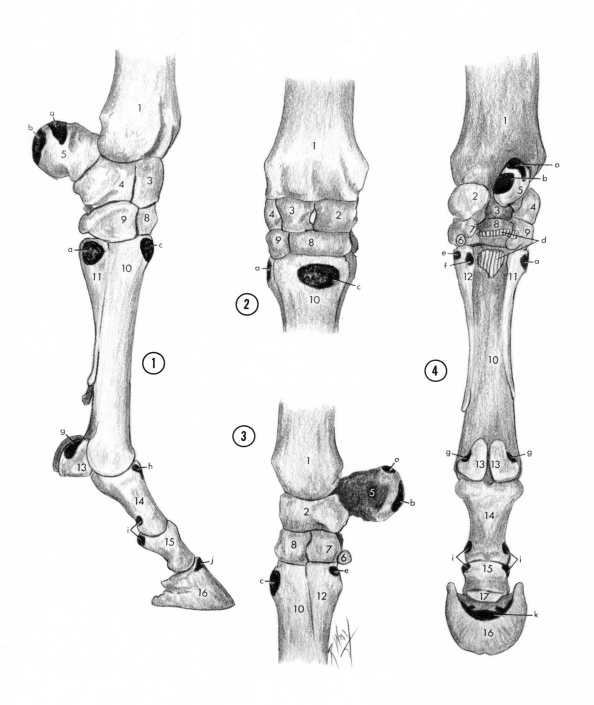

(Plate 34)   77

SECTION SIX

The Pectoral Region and the Front Limb

PLATE 35

The cutaneous nerves of the shoulder region and the lateral aspect of the front limb

1. Medial dorsal branches of the 7th and the 8th cervical nerves
2. Medial dorsal branches of the first 10 thoracic nerves
3. Lateral dorsal branches of thoracic nerves
4. Superficial branches of ventral thoracic nerves
5. Intercostobrachial nerve, which is the lateral cutaneous branch of the 2nd intercostal nerve
6. Lateral ventral branch of the 6th cervical nerve
7. Cranial cutaneous antebrachial branch of the axillary nerve
8. Lateral cutaneous antebrachial branch of the radial nerve
9. Caudal cutaneous antebrachial branch of the ulnar nerve
10. Dorsal branch of the ulnar nerve
11. A branch of the medial cutaneous antebrachial from the musculocutaneous nerve
12. Anastomotic branch connecting the medial and the lateral volar metacarpal nerves
13. Lateral volar metacarpal nerve formed by the union above the carpus of the lateral branch of the median nerve and the volar branch of the ulnar nerve.

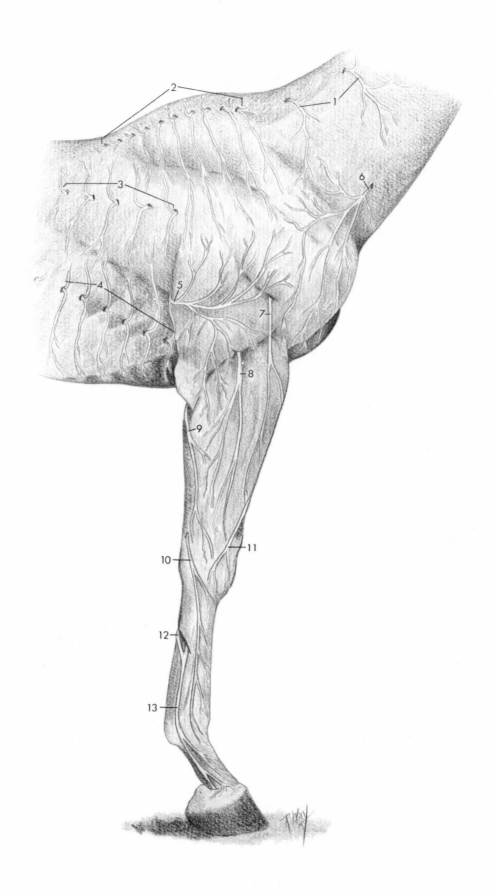

(Plate 35)   81

PLATE 36

The muscles which attach the front limb to the trunk and the superficial muscles of the lateral aspect of the front limb.

Muscles 1 to 9 serve to attach the limb to the trunk. There is no bony articulation between the front limb and the bones of the trunk, since the clavicle is reduced to a fibrous band in the substance of the brachiocephalic muscle (cleido-mastoideus).

1. The brachiocephalic muscle, which extends from the head and the neck to the lateral aspect of the humerus to insert on the deltoid tuberosity and the crest
2. Cervical portion of the serratus ventralis muscle, extending from the transverse process of the last 4 cervical vertebrae to the inner surface of the scapula
3. & 4. Cervical portion (3) and thoracic portion (4) of the trapezius muscle. This arises dorsally from the supraspinous ligament and converges distally to insert on the spine of the scapula.
5. Latissimus dorsi muscle
6. Thoracic part of the serratus ventralis muscle. Only a small portion is visible. This arises from the lateral surfaces of the first 8 or 9 ribs and extends dorsally to insert on the medial aspect of the scapula.
7. Cranial deep pectoral muscle
8. Caudal deep pectoral muscle
9. Cranial superficial pectoral muscle
10. Deltoideus muscle, arising from the spine and the caudal border of the scapula and inserting below on the deltoid truberosity
11 & 12. Long head (11) and lateral head (12) of the triceps brachii muscle. The long head arises from the caudal border of the scapula, whereas the lateral head arises from the deltoid tuberosity of the humerus. Both heads insert on the olecranon process of the ulna.
13. Extensor carpi radialis, arising above from the lateral condyloid crest of the humerus and inserting below on the metacarpal tuberosity
14. Common digital extensor, which arises from the lateral distal surface of the humerus and the lateral tuberosity and border of the radius. Its long tendon extends downward over the carpus and metacarpus to insert chiefly on the extensor process of the 3rd phalanx.
15. Lateral digital extensor, which arises from the lateral tuberosity and border of the radius and the shaft of the ulna. Its tendon is at first small but, below the carpus, receives a branch from the common extensor and a strong band from the accessory carpal bone. These contributions result in enlarging the tendon to a broad flat band. This extends distally to insert on the front of the proximal extremity of the first phalanx.
16. Ulnaris lateralis muscle, arising from the lateral epicondyle of the humerus and inserting on the accessory carpal bone and the lateral or 4th metacarpal
17. Ulnar head of the deep digital flexor
18. Extensor carpi obliquus muscle, which curves obliquely over the carpus. It arises from the lateral border of the radius and its long tendon inserts on the head of the medial or 2nd metacarpal bone.

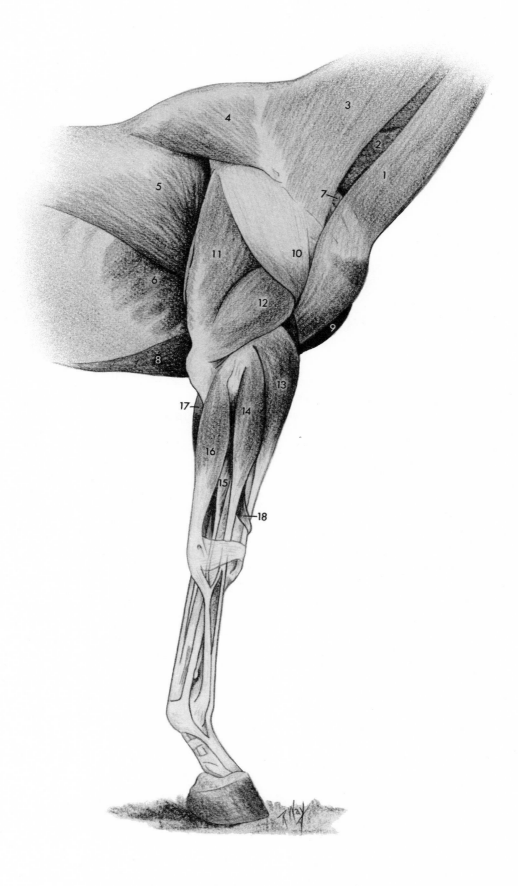

(Plate 36) 83

PLATE 37

The deeper muscles attaching the front limb to the trunk. The brachiocephalicus and the cervical and thoracic portions of the trapezius have been removed.

1. The rhomboideus muscle, which arises from the supraspinous ligament and inserts on the medial aspect of the scapular cartilage

2. & 3. Thoracic portion (2) and cervical portion (3) of the serratus ventralis muscle
4. Superficial cervical or prescapular lymph nodes, which are covered by the brachiocephalic muscle
5. Cranial deep pectoral muscle
6. Supraspinatus muscle
7. Distal end of the infraspinatus muscle
8. Deltoideus muscle
9. & 10. Long head (9) and lateral head (10) of the triceps brachii muscle
11. Biceps brachii muscle, proximal end
12. Cut edge of the brachiocephalicus

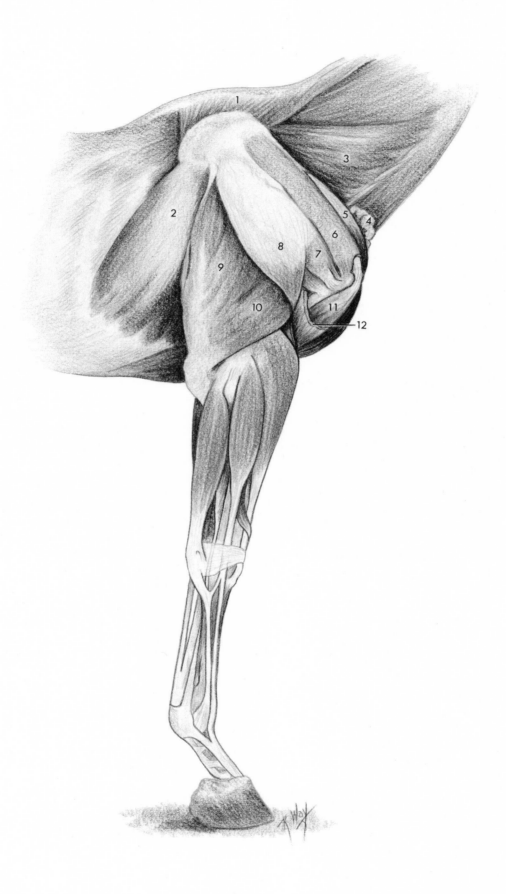

(Plate 37)   85

PLATE 38

The deep muscles of the shoulder, the arm and the forearm

1. Supraspinatus muscle, arising from the spine and the supraspinous fossa of the scapula and inserting on the cranial portions of both the medial and the lateral tuberosities of the humerus
2. Infraspinatus muscle, arising from the infraspinous fossa and inserting on the lateral tuberosity of the humerus
3. Teres minor muscle, which arises from the caudal border of the scapula and inserts on the deltoid tuberosity of the humerus and an area just above it
4. Brachialis muscle, which arises from the proximal third of the caudal surface of the humerus and spirals laterally over the lateral surface of the humerus (following the contour of the musculo-spiral groove) to reach the medial surface of the elbow. It inserts on the proximal end of the medial surface of the radius.
5. Proximal end of the biceps brachii muscle
6. Cranial deep pectoral muscle
7. Anconeus muscle, which arises from the distal third of the caudal surface of the humerus and inserts on the olecranon
8. Extensor carpi obliquus muscle
9. Ulnaris lateralis muscle

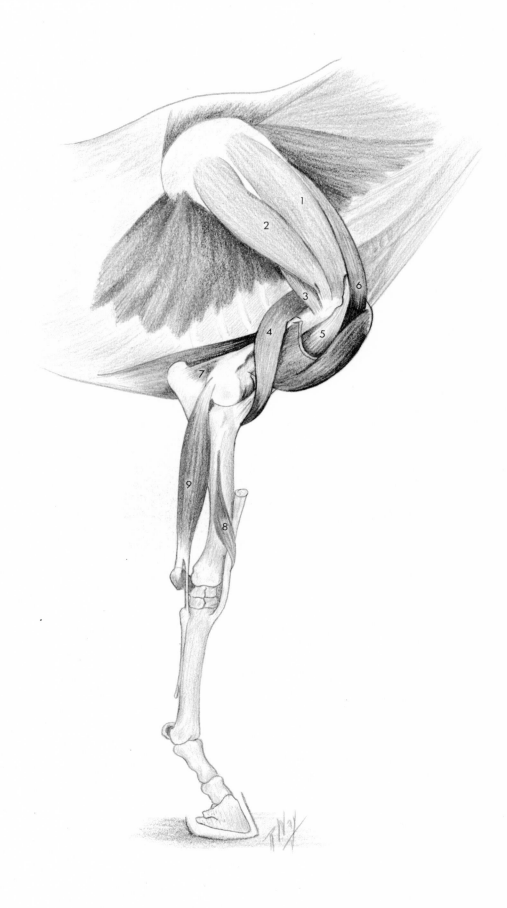

(Plate 38) 87

PLATE 39

The deepest muscles of the shoulder and the arm

1. Rhomboideus muscle
2. & 3. Thoracic (2) and cervical (3) portions of the serratus ventralis muscle
4. Cranial deep pectoral muscle
5. Teres minor muscle, which arises from the lower part of the infraspinous fossa and posterior border of the scapula and inserts on a small area above the deltoid tuberosity of the humerus
6. Tendon of origin of the biceps brachii
7. Tendon of insertion of the biceps brachii
8. Caudal deep pectoral muscle
9. & 10. Lateral digital extensor (9) and its tendon (10)
11. Proximal end of the brachialis muscle
12. Stump of the brachiocephalicus muscle, which has dropped downward
13. Stump of the cranial superficial pectoral muscle
14. Flap of the cutaneous omobrachialis

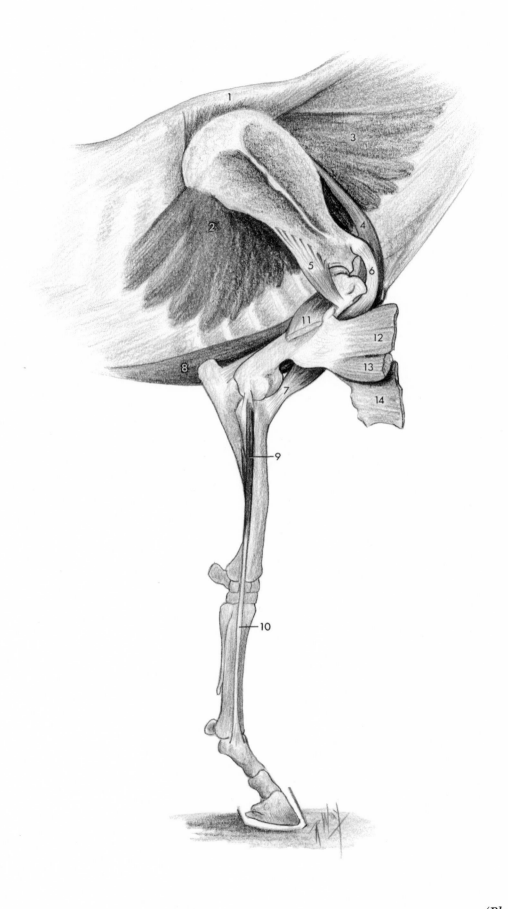

(Plate 39)   89

PLATE 40

The latissimus dorsi and the deep pectoral muscles

1. Latissimus dorsi muscle, arising dorsally from the supraspinous ligament by means of a broad, flat aponeurosis and extending distally to insert on the teres tuberosity of the humerus

2. Caudal deep pectoral muscle, which arises from the cartilages of ribs 4 to 9, the ventral aspect of the sternum, and the abdominal tunic. It inserts chiefly on the cranial portion of the medial tuberosity of the humerus.
3. Cranial deep pectoral muscle arising from the cranial half of the lateral surface of the sternum and the first 4 costal cartilages. It inserts on the cranial border of the scapula.

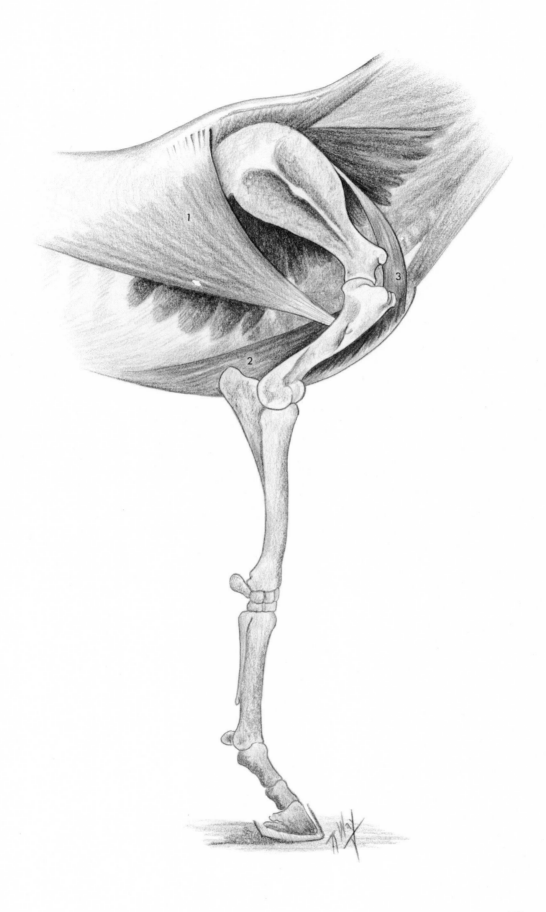

(Plate 40)   91

PLATE 41

A view of the cranial surface of the pectoral region, the shoulder and the arm. Superficial dissection.

1. Cutaneous colli muscle, which arises from the cariniform cartilage of the sternum
2. Brachiocephalicus muscle
3. Cranial superficial pectoral muscle, which arises from the cariniform cartilage of the sternum and inserts on the deltoid tuberosity of the humerus
4. Caudal superficial pectoral muscle, which arises from the ventral edge of the sternum and inserts on the curved line of the humerus and fascia of the forearm
5. Distal end of the biceps brachii muscle
6. Distal end of the brachialis muscle. The aponeurosis of the brachiocephalicus, which extends to the fascia covering the extensor carpi radialis, has been removed to make (5) and (6) visible.
7. Medial cutaneous antebrachial nerve, derived from the musculocutaneous nerve
8. Cranial cutaneous antebrachial nerve, derived from the axillary nerve
9. Cephalic vein, which arises at the medial side of the carpus as the upward continuation of the medial volar metacarpal vein and terminates above, either by opening into the terminal end of the jugular vein or into the axillary vein
10. Accessory cephalic vein, which arises at the carpus and joins the cephalic vein at the proximal end of the forearm
11. Extensor carpi radialis muscle
12. Radius, here covered only by skin and fascia
13. Flexor carpi radialis muscle

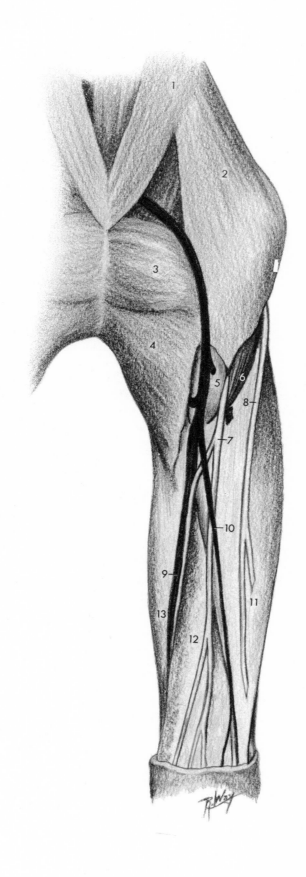

(Plate 41) 93

PLATE 42

The muscles of the front limb as viewed from the medial surface

1. & 2. Rhomboideus cervicalis (1) and thoracalis (2) muscles
3. Latissimus dorsi muscle
4. Teres major muscle, arising from the caudal border of the scapula and inserting in common with the tendon of the latissimus dorsi on the teres tuberosity of the humerus
5. Subscapularis muscle, originating from the subscapular fossa and inserting on the caudal eminence of the medial tuberosity of the humerus
6. Supraspinatus muscle
7. Stump of the cranial deep pectoral muscle
8. Stump of the caudal deep pectoral muscle
9. Biceps brachii muscle
10. The coracobrachialis muscle, which arises from the coracoid process of the scapula and inserts on the cranial surface of the humerus at the middle third
11. Medial head of the triceps brachii, which arises from the medial surface of the humerus below the teres tuberosity and inserts on the olecranon process of the ulna
12. Tensor fasciae antebrachii muscle, which arises mainly from the tendon of insertion of the latissimus dorsi and inserts on the deep antebrachial fascia and olecranon
13. Flexor carpi ulnaris muscle. Note that, above, it has two heads of origin—ulnar and humeral. The ulnar head arises from the medial surface of the olecranon. The humeral head arises from the medial epicondyle of the humerus. The muscle inserts on the accessory carpal bone.
14. Flexor carpi radialis muscle, which arises from the medial epicondyle of the humerus and inserts on the proximal end of the second metacarpal
15. Radius
16. Extensor carpi radialis muscle
17. Tendon of the extensor carpi obliquus muscle

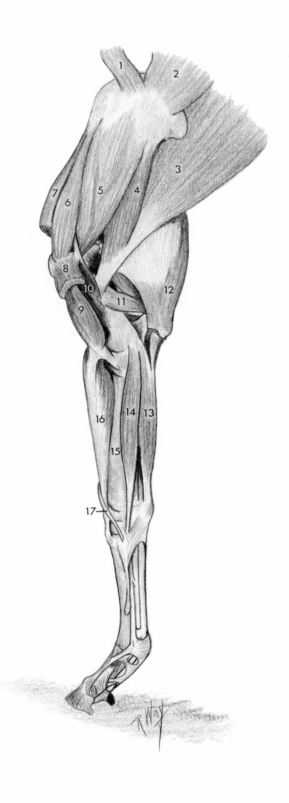

(Plate 42) 95

PLATE 43

A deeper dissection of the muscles of the arm and forearm regions as viewed from the medial surface

1. Coracobrachialis muscle
2. Biceps brachii muscle
3. Insertion of the brachialis muscle
4. Humeral head of the superficial digital flexor, arising from the medial epicondyle of the humerus
5. Radial head of the superficial digital flexor, a strong fibrous band often termed the superior check ligament, since it checks or prevents flexion of the carpus during sleep in the standing position

6. Medial insertion of the tendon of the superficial digital flexor. Near its end the tendon bifurcates and inserts on the medial and the lateral surfaces of the distal end of the first and the proximal end of the second phalanges.
7. Ulnar head of the deep digital flexor
8. Humeral head of the deep digital flexor
9. Tendon of the deep digital flexor
10. Inferior check ligament, which aids the superior check ligament in fixing the carpus during sleep. It arises from the volar ligament of the carpus and joins the tendon of the deep flexor about the middle of the metacarpal region.
11. The end of the deep flexor tendon which inserts on the semilunar crest of the 3rd phalanx
12. Interosseous medius, which in the horse, is almost entirely tendinous and is frequently termed the suspensory ligament of the fetlock

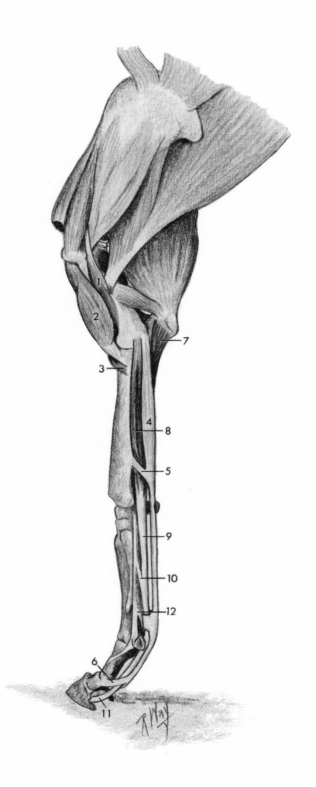

(Plate 43)   97

PLATE 44

Special dissection of the deep muscles of the arm region and of the deep digital flexor, viewed from the medial side

1. & 2. Brachialis muscle
3. Coracobrachialis muscle
4. Biceps brachii muscle, which originates from the scapular tuberosity and inserts on the radial tuberosity
5. Long head of the triceps brachii
6, 7, 8, & 9. Ulnar head (6), humeral head (7), radial head (8) and tendon (9) of the deep digital flexor. The ulnar head arises from the medial surface of the olecranon, the humeral head from the medial epicondyle, and the radial head from the middle of the caudal surface of the radius.
10. Inferior check ligament
11. Suspensory ligament of the fetlock

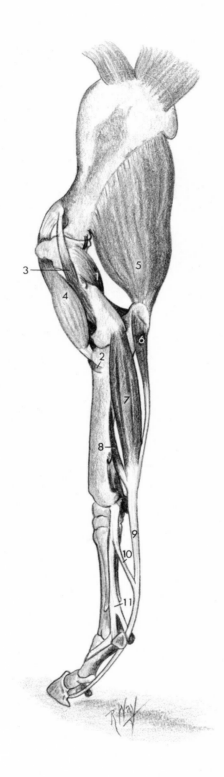

(Plate 44)   99

PLATE 45

Figure 1. Illustrating the arrangement of the major arteries in relation to the bones of the front limb.

Medial view:

1. Axillary
2. Suprascapular
3. Subscapular
4. Circumflex scapular
5. Thoracodorsal
6. Caudal circumflex humeral
7. Cranial circumflex humeral
8. Deep brachial
9. Brachial
10. Collateral ulnar
11. Median
12. Distal collateral radial
13. Common interosseous
14. Artery of rete carpi volare
15. Lateral deep volar metacarpal
16. Medial deep volar metacarpal

17. Medial superficial volar metacarpal or common digital

Figure 2. Illustrating the arrangement of the major veins in relation to the bones of the front limb.

Medial view:

1. Jugular
2. Axillary
3. Suprascapular
4. Circumflex scapular
5. Subscapular
6. Caudal circumflex humeral
7. Thoracodorsal
8. Cranial circumflex humeral
9. Brachial
10. Deep brachial
11. Collateral ulnar
12. Cephalic
13. Medial cubital
14. Median
15. Accessory cephalic
16. Lateral volar metacarpal
17. Deep volar metacarpal
18. Medial volar metacarpal

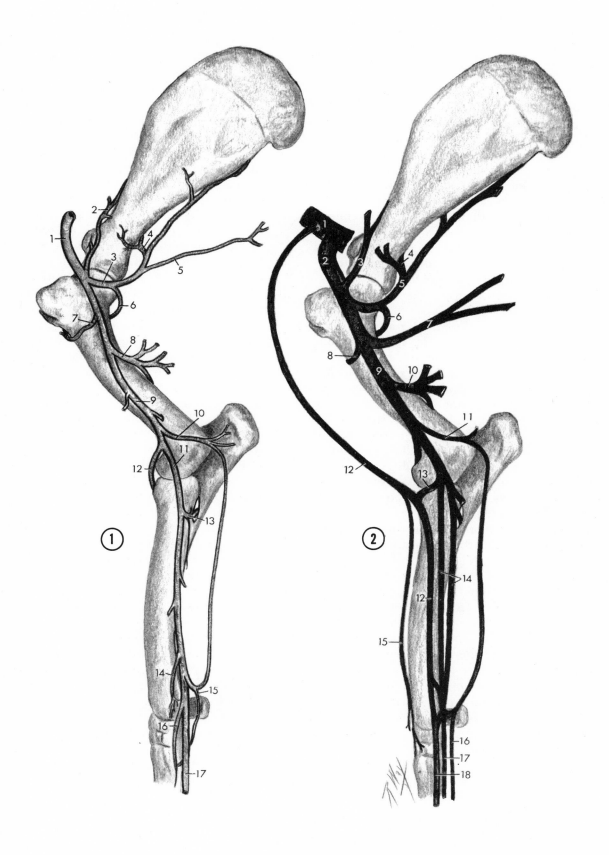

(Plate 45)   101

PLATE 46

Deep dissection of the lateral surface of the shoulder and arm regions. The long and the lateral heads of the triceps brachii muscle have been cut and reflected caudally; the teres minor and the deltoideus have been cut and reflected ventrally together. The supraspinatus and the infraspinatus muscles have been transected near their insertions and the remainder of their substance has been stripped from their respective fossae.

1. Terminal branch of the subscapular artery, running over the dorsal part of the infraspinous fossa and helping to supply the infraspinatus muscle
2. Stump of the deltoideus muscle, arising from the caudal angle of the scapula, and the stump of the teres major just cranial to it
3. Latissimus dorsi muscle, being medial to the aponeurosis of the tensor fasciae antebrachii and joining with the tendon of teres major
4. The thin, aponeurotic origin of the tensor fasciae antebrachii muscle from the caudal border of the scapula, and the contiguous tendon of the teres major cranially
5. Subscapular vein, running caudal to the artery
6. Subscapular artery, situated behind the caudal border of the scapula
7. Some of the fibers of origin of the triceps brachii muscle, arising from the caudal border of the scapula
8. Lateral branch of the circumflex artery of the scapula, running around the neck of the scapula
9. Suprascapular nerve, crossing over the cranial border of the scapula to innervate the supraspinatus and the infraspinatus muscles
10. Tendon of origin of the biceps brachii muscle from the tuber scapulae
11. Insertion of the supraspinatus onto the cranial part of the lateral tuberosity of the humerus; this muscle bridges over the tendon of origin of the biceps to insert onto the cranial part of the medial tuberosity.
12. Head of the humerus, capped by the glenoid cavity of the scapula
13. The small, fusiform capsularis muscle just behind the capsule of the shoulder joint, arising from the scapula and inserting between the muscular fibers of the brachialis
14. Axillary nerve, running laterally with the caudal humeral circumflex artery behind the shoulder joint. Its muscular branches can be seen entering the lateral head of the triceps. Another branch (which was cut short) innervates the brachiocephalicus muscle. The long branch is the cranial cutaneous antebrachial nerve derived from the axillary.
15. Deeply placed brachialis muscle lying in the musculospiral groove of the humerus
16. The large radial nerve emerging just caudal to the tendon of insertion of the teres major muscle. The large branch (which is cut short) innervates the long head of the triceps brachii muscle. The superficial branches lying over the extensor carpi radialis muscle are the cutaneous branches of the radial nerve.
17. Artery running between the radial nerve and the vein. This is a branch of the deep brachial artery and the corresponding large vein is the deep brachial vein.
18. Origin of the lateral head of the triceps from the curved line on the humerus which runs from the deltoid tuberosity upward toward the head
19. Circular area on the tendon of insertion of the infraspinatus muscle. This represents the bursa between this long tendon of insertion and the caudal part of the lateral tuberosity. The short fibers of insertion of the infraspinatus muscle can be seen inserting directly on the caudal part of the lateral tuberosity, just cranial to (12).
20. Hanging deltoideus muscle, attached to the deltoid tuberosity of the humerus
21. Brachiocephalicus muscle, hanging under the deltoideus muscle
22. Origin of the extensor carpi radialis from the lateral condyloid crest of the humerus
23. Anconeus muscle, lying over the olecranon fossa

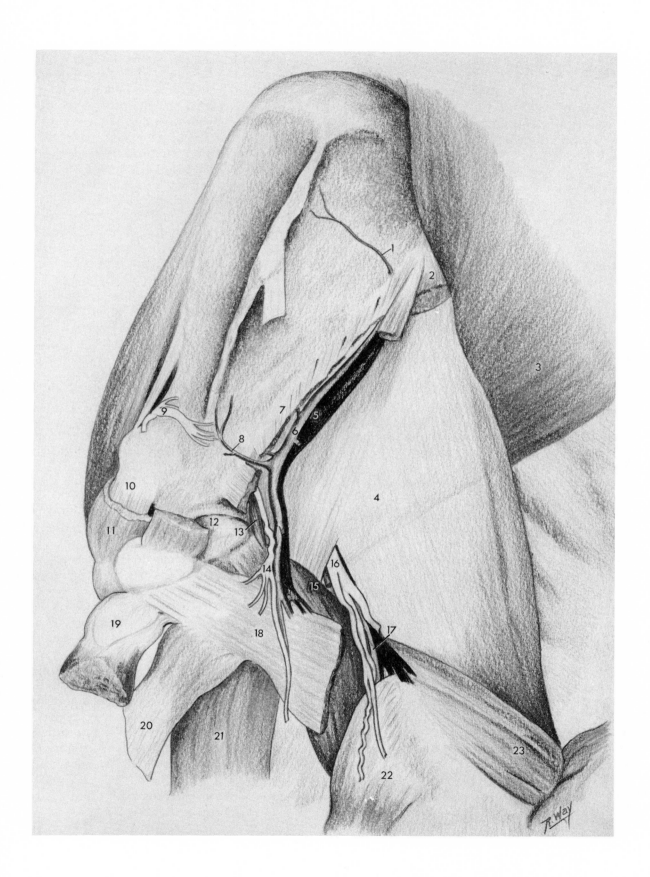

(Plate 46) 103

PLATE 47

The lateral surface of the brachial and the proximal portions of the antebrachial regions. Deep dissection.

1. Suprascapular nerve, winding around the lower part of the cranial border of the scapula to reach the lateral aspect and protected by a connective tissue bridge
2. Lateral branch of the circumflex scapular artery, emerging between the fibers of origin of the long head of the triceps brachii muscle at the caudal part of the neck of the scapula
3. Axillary nerve, reaching the lateral aspect (in company with the caudal circumflex humeral artery) just behind the shoulder joint
4. The small, cranial twig of the caudal circumflex humeral artery running over the lateral and the cranial surfaces of the humerus to join the cranial circumflex humeral artery
5. The supraspinatus muscle has been entirely freed from its insertions onto the dorsal parts of the cranial portions of both tuberosities of the humerus.
6. Origin of the lateral head of the triceps brachii muscle
7. Bursa, overlying the caudal part of the lateral tuberosity of the humerus beneath the long tendon of insertion of the infraspinatus muscle
8. Origin of the biceps brachii muscle from the tuber scapulae. Note the groove in its tendon, which has been reflected.
9. Aponeurotic insertion of the caudal deep pectoral muscle onto the lip of the cranial part of the lateral tuberosity of the humerus
10. The heavy, tendinous insertion (cross-hatched) of the long tendon of the infraspinatus muscle onto the roughened area behind the cranial and below the caudal parts of the lateral tuberosity of the humerus
11. Portion of the teres minor muscle, attached to the lateral surface of the humerus just cranial to the deltoid tuberosity
12. Deltoid tuberosity, with a tag of the deltoideus muscle attached to it
13. Common sheet of insertion of the brachiocephalicus and the superficial pectoral muscles attached to the lower part of the deltoid tuberosity and to the crest of the humerus
14. Spirally shaped brachialis muscle occupying the musculospiral groove of the humerus
15. Radial nerve (in company with the deep brachial artery) running behind the caudal border of the brachialis muscle to reach the front of the elbow where it then travels caudally to reach the ulnaris lateralis muscle in company with the distal collateral radial artery. To expose the latter, the extensor carpi radialis and the common digital extensor muscles have been cut at their origins and reflected downward.
16. Extensor carpi radialis, arising from the lateral condyloid crest of the humerus and, lower down (16'), the origins of the common digital extensor from the lateral collateral ligament of the elbow and the lateral tuberosity of the radius
17. Origin of the long head of the triceps brachii muscle from the caudal border of the scapula
18. Anconeus muscle, inserting on the craniolateral surface of the olecranon of the ulna
19. Portion of the ulnar head of the deep digital flexor muscle
20. Origin of the ulnaris lateralis from the lateral epicondyle of the humerus
21. Origin of the lateral digital extensor muscle from the lateral tuberosity of the radius and the lateral ligament of the elbow
22. Tendon of the biceps brachii muscle, just above the distal part of the brachialis, inserting onto the radial tuberosity
23. The vertically descending branch of the distal collateral radial artery, which receives an anastomotic branch from the common interosseous artery
24. Common interosseous artery, emerging under the lateral digital extensor muscle to descend vertically and send over the aforementioned anastomotic branch. It then continues downward as the dorsal interosseous artery. The dorsal interosseous and the anterior radial arteries contribute to the formation of the rete carpi dorsale.
25. Origin of the extensor carpi obliquus from the lateral border of the radius

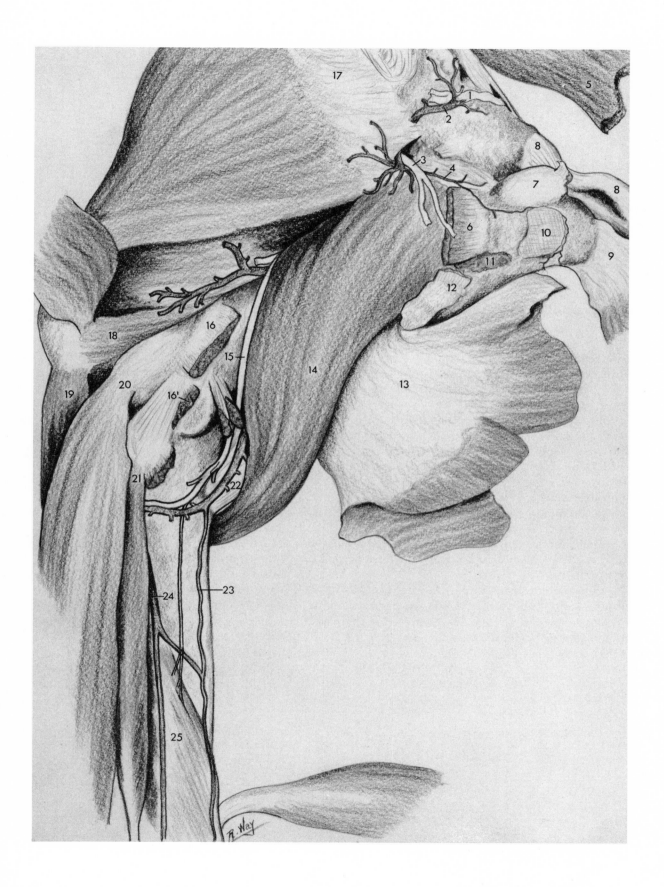

(Plate 47)   105

PLATE 48

The brachial plexus. The pectoral muscles and the brachiocephalic muscle have been cut and the limb abducted with the horse in an upright position.

In the horse, the brachial plexus is formed by the ventral branches of the last three cervical and the first two thoracic spinal nerves.

1. & 2. Small dorsal part (1) and large ventral part (2) of the scalenus muscle, between which the major branches of the last three cervical nerves emerge
3. Ventral branch of the 6th cervical nerve bifurcating to send one branch downward over the scalenus muscle as the chief root of the phrenic nerve. The dorsal branch enters the brachial plexus.
4. Ventral branch of the 7th cervical nerve
5. Ventral branch of the 8th cervical nerve
6. A branch from the 7th cervical which joins with a branch from the 6th to form the phrenic nerve
7. Pectoral nerve cut when the pectoral muscles were reflected
8. The musculocutaneous nerve, formed by contributions from the 6th, the 7th, and the 8th cervical nerves. It passes downward over the surface of the scalenus muscle lateral to the axillary artery and joins the median nerve.

9. A branch of the musculocutaneous nerve which supplies the biceps brachii muscle
10. Confluence of the axillary and the jugular veins
11. Axillary artery
12. The long thoracic nerve, formed by branches from the 7th and the 8th cervicals, which emerge through the dorsal part of the scalenus muscle. This nerve supplies branches to the serratus ventralis muscle.
13. Thoracodorsal nerve, which supplies the latissimus dorsi muscle
14. Subscapular nerve, which supplies the subscapularis muscle
15. Suprascapular nerve, derived from the 6th and the 7th cervicals, which supplies the supraspinatus and the infraspinatus muscles
16. External thoracic nerve, which supplies branches to the caudal deep pectoral muscle, the cutaneous trunci muscle and the skin of the ventral thoracic wall
17. Axillary nerve, derived chiefly from the 8th cervical
18. Radial nerve, derived chiefly from the 1st thoracic nerve
19. Ulnar nerve, derived from the thoracic components of the plexus
20. Median nerve, derived chiefly from the first thoracic nerve. Note the loop formed under the brachial artery by the musculocutaneous which joins the median.

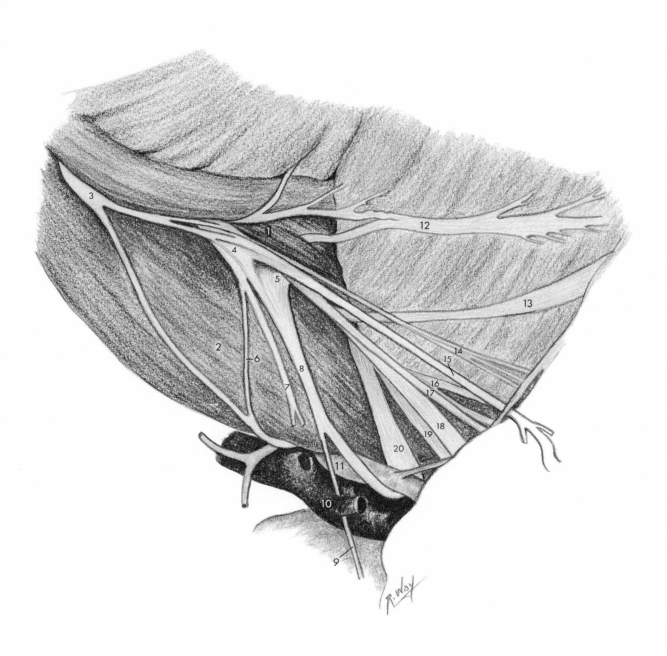

(Plate 48)   107

PLATE 49

The medial surface of the shoulder and the arm after removal from the body. The following muscles have been cut: the superficial pectorals, the brachiocephalicus, the deep pectorals, the omohyoideus, and the serratus ventralis.

1. Suprascapular nerve, disappearing between the supraspinatus and the subscapularis muscles
2. Subscapular nerves, innervating the subscapularis muscle
3. Axillary nerve, disappearing between the subscapularis and the teres major muscles in company with the subscapular artery and vein
4. The branch from the axillary nerve which innervates the teres major muscle

5. Thoracodorsal nerve, extending back to supply the latissimus dorsi muscle
6. Musculocutaneous nerve, cranial in position, crossing the lateral surface of the axillary artery and helping to form the loop under the artery with the median nerve
7. Median nerve crossing the medial face of the artery, joining the musculocutaneous and descending cranial to the artery in the medial brachial region. Note the branch (7a) which leaves the median at the caudal limitation of the coracobrachialis and just dorsal to the biceps brachii to disappear under cover of that muscle. This is the medial cutaneous antebrachial branch of the musculocutaneous nerve. Note the median nerve crossing the artery (and under the median cubital vein) to become caudal to the artery at the elbow.
8. Ulnar nerve, just caudal to the median and closely adherent to the large radial nerve. It

runs under cover of the brachial vein but reappears a little lower down and then disappears under cover of the tensor fasciae antebrachii muscle. A branch of the ulnar nerve, the caudal cutaneous antebrachial branch (8a), continues downward along the cranial border of the tensor fasciae antebrachii muscle to curve around the caudal part of the elbow and ramify on both surfaces of the caudal part of the forearm.

9. Large radial nerve running with the ulnar. However, the brachial vein covers the area where it disappears between the muscles. This can be seen in the next illustration.

10. The external thoracic nerve can be seen running directly backward.

11. Axillary artery, suspended in the loop formed by the musculocutaneous and the median nerves. It then descends obliquely downward and backward as the brachial artery between the median nerve cranially and the brachial vein caudally.

12. Suprascapular artery, arising from the axillary, ascending over the subscapularis muscle, sending twigs into the supraspinatus and disappearing in the cleft between those two muscles in company with the suprascapular nerve

13. Large subscapular artery, arising from the axillary and disappearing almost immediately between the subscapularis and the teres major muscles in company with the axillary nerve. However, before disappearing, it gives rise to the thoracodorsal artery (13a) which can be seen running caudally to supply the latissimus dorsi muscle.

14. In the middle of the arm the large deep brachial artery, arising from the brachial, is almost completely covered caudally by the brachial vein. It is seen to better advantage in the next illustration.

(Plate 49)   109

15. Ulnar artery, arising from the brachial just dorsal to the cubital lymph nodes and then being covered by the brachial vein and the tensor fasciae antebrachii muscle. It is better illustrated in the next plate.
16. Large brachial vein, ascending behind the brachial artery in the brachial region
17. Large thoracodorsal vein entering the brachial. The external thoracic vein (cut) can be seen joining the thoracodorsal and entering the brachial by a common trunk.
18. The oblique branch, the median cubital vein, which is given off from the cephalic and helps to form the brachial.
19. Observe a deep median vein and two superficial ones, which drain the flexor muscles, entering the median cubital vein.
20. Axillary lymph node, caudal to the brachial and dorsal to the thoracodorsal veins

21. Cubital lymph node, just ventral to the origin of the ulnar artery
22. Insertion of the cranial deep pectoral muscle onto the dorsal part of the cranial border of the scapula
23. Omohyoideus muscle, arising from the subscapular fascia
24. The supraspinatus, inserting onto the cranial part of the medial tuberosity of the humerus
25. Caudal deep pectoral muscle, inserting onto the medial tuberosity and sending an aponeurosis over to the lateral tuberosity of the humerus
26. Latissimus dorsi, coming downward and forward to insert with the teres major
27. Tensor fasciae antebrachii muscle, covering the medial and the long heads of the triceps brachii and inserting onto the fascia of the forearm

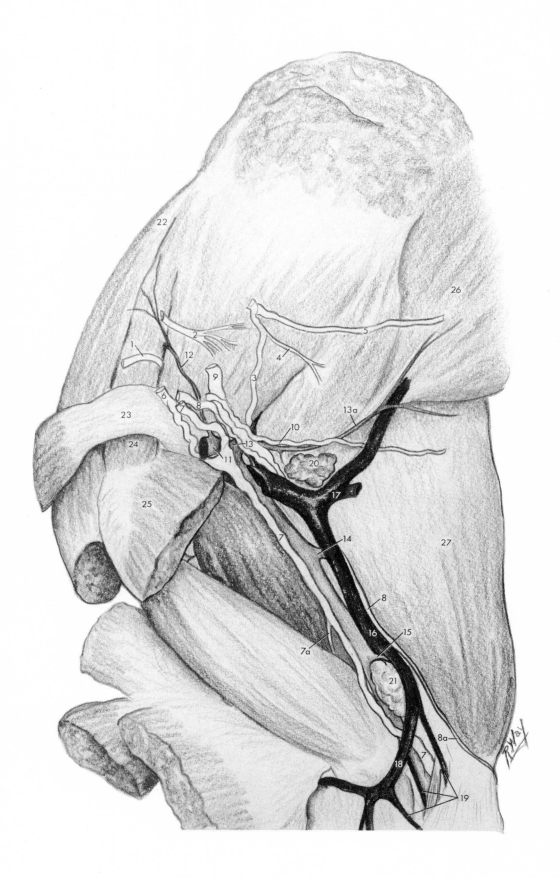

(Plate 49)   111

PLATE 50

The medial surface of the shoulder and the arm—deep dissection.

In addition to the procedures carried out for the preparation of Plate 49, the following was done: the omohyoideus was transected, leaving only a small tag; the supraspinatus muscle was cut from its insertion onto the cranial part of the medial tuberosity and reflected cranio-laterally; the caudal deep pectoral muscle was cut (and reflected laterally) from its insertion onto the tendon of the coracobrachialis and the lip of the cranial part of the medial tuberosity, leaving a tag; the tensor fasciae antebrachii has been removed, and a considerable portion of the brachial vessels (and the median nerve) was removed in order to show the collateral branches.

1. Axillary nerve and subscapular artery and vein disappearing between the subscapularis and the teres major muscles. The thoracodorsal artery can be seen arising from the subscapular artery.
2. Radial nerve and deep brachial artery and vein disappearing together between the long and the medial heads of the triceps brachii muscle
3. Ulnar nerve, running over the medial head of the triceps brachii muscle, then under (lateral to) the collateral ulnar vein and artery to descend with these vessels under cover of the flexor carpi ulnaris muscle. Note the branch of the ulnar nerve descending to innervate the flexor carpi ulnaris, and the branch of the collateral ulnar artery which runs over the medial epicondyle of the humerus to supply the tensor fasciae antebrachii muscle. (It was, of course, cut when the muscle was removed.)
4. The tiny, fusiform muscle which arises from the medial collateral ligament of the elbow and binds down somewhat the median nerve and vessels and then inserts onto the lower part of the ligament. This is the pronator teres muscle.
5. Origin of the flexor carpi radialis muscle from the medial epicondyle of the humerus, just cranial to the origin of the flexor carpi ulnaris muscle
6. Origin of the flexor carpi ulnaris muscle from the medial epicondyle of the humerus and from the olecranon of the ulna
7. Subcutaneous medial border of the radius and the cephalic and accessory cephalic veins
8. Tendon of insertion of the biceps brachii muscle, merging with the tendon of the extensor carpi radialis and inserting caudally onto the medial collateral ligament of the elbow.
9. The small portion of the brachialis muscle which is visible just ventral to the tendon of the biceps and in front of the medial collateral ligament of the elbow.
10. Medial head of the triceps brachii inserting onto the medial surface of the olecranon
11. Conjoined aponeurosis of the brachiocephalicus and the superficial pectoral muscles inserting onto the crest of the humerus
12. Tendon of origin of the biceps brachii from the tuber scapulae
13. Tendon of origin of the coracobrachialis from the coracoid process

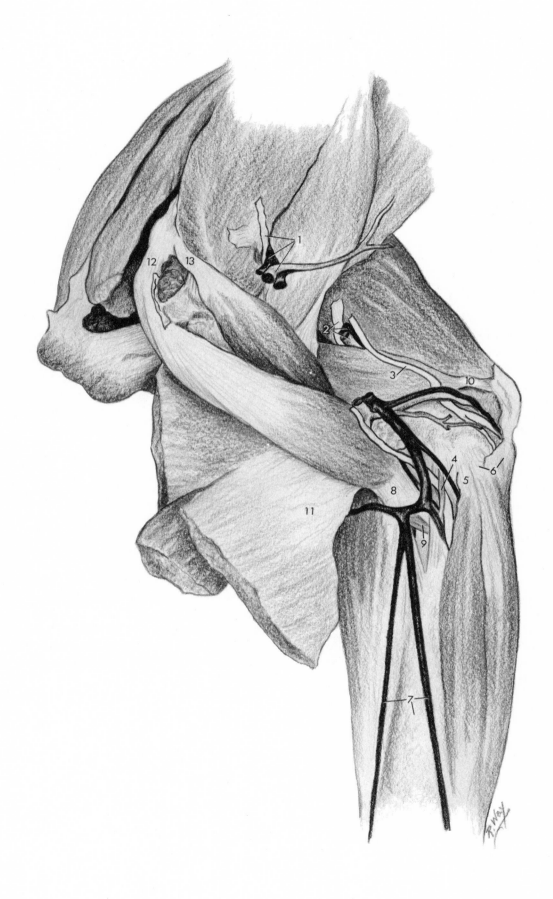

(Plate 50)   113

PLATE 51

The medial surface of the forearm or the antebrachial region. The antebrachial fascia has been removed; the flexor carpi radialis muscle has been incised in its ventral tendinous portion and the upper portion has been reflected dorsally.

1. Median nerve, crossing behind the artery at the elbow, then crossing a little further down to become cranial (under cover of the muscle). Here it gives off a large branch to the deep flexor and a couple of smaller twigs to the flexor carpi radialis. Lower down, it inclines caudally and terminates above the carpus. Note the lateral terminal branch above the lateral deep volar metacarpal artery.
2. Median artery, crossing the medial collateral ligament of the elbow. It then dips under (lateral to) the flexor carpi radialis muscle which has been reflected to show the vessels and the nerve. The artery descends vertically, giving off twigs to the flexors.
3. Artery of the rete carpi volare, arising from the distal part of the median
4. Medial deep volar metacarpal artery, running downward in company with the cephalic vein
5. Lateral deep volar metacarpal artery running caudally above a vein and below a nerve
6. The accessory cephalic and the cephalic veins. Note the branch in the carpal region that runs caudally to give origin to the two median veins.

7. In the proximal region, the three median veins; one joining the median cubital vein close to the entrance of the cephalic; the middle one *deep* in position and ascending cranial to the artery, and the third one entering the median cubital in its proximal portion. Another deep median vein which runs behind the artery cannot be seen. However, the deep veins can be seen joining the median cubital immediately above the origin of the ulnar artery to form the brachial vein. The collateral ulnar vein also can be seen joining the median cubital and helping to form the brachial vein.
8. Biceps brachii muscle, inserting on the medial collateral ligament of the elbow joint and tendon of the extensor carpi radialis muscle.
9. Small pronator teres muscle
10. Tendon of insertion of the flexor carpi radialis muscle
11. Reflected deep layer of the antebrachial fascia
12. Origin of the flexor carpi radialis muscle from the medial epicondyle of the humerus
13. Origin of the humeral head of the flexor carpi ulnaris muscle—just behind the preceding (12), from the medial epicondyle of the humerus. Note, also, the origin of the ulnar head from the olecranon and the blending distally of the two heads.
14. Cubital lymph node, dorsal to the median cubital vein and ventral to the origin of the collateral ulnar artery and overlying the median artery

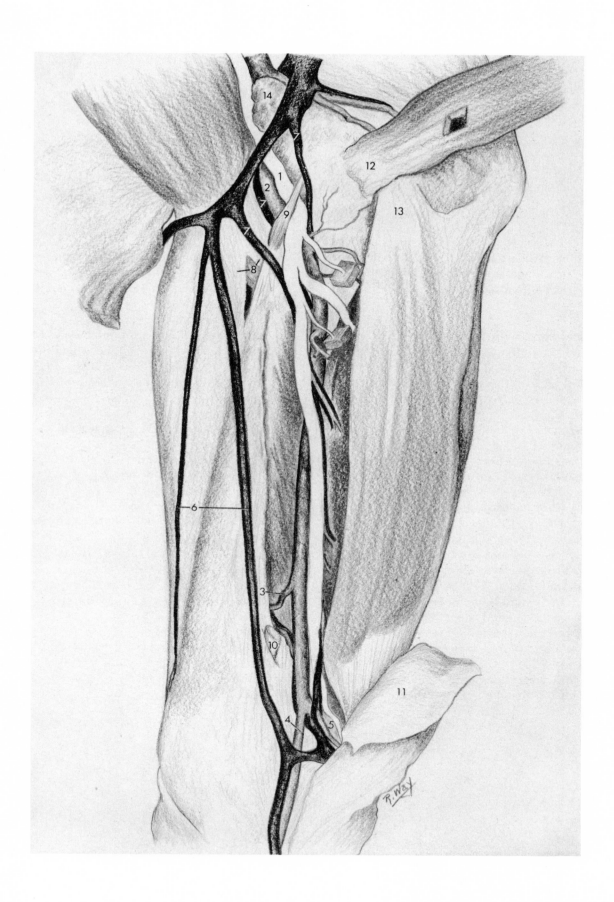

(Plate 51)   115

PLATE 52

The medial surface of the carpus and the digit. The flexor carpi radialis muscle has been removed and the flexor carpi ulnaris muscle reflected caudally.

1. Median artery, with the cephalic vein cranial to it and, caudally, a median vein and the median nerve
2. Humeral head of the superficial digital flexor
3. Ulnar vein and nerve. These are accompanied by the ulnar artery which lies under (lateral to) the vein.
4. Distal end of the flexor carpi ulnaris muscle, which has been reflected caudally
5. Distal end of the extensor carpi radialis muscle
6. Tendon of the extensor carpi obliquus muscle
7. Artery of the rete carpi volare, branching off the median artery. In this specimen the medial deep volar metacarpal artery branched from the artery of the rete and can be seen going distad behind the cephalic vein.
8. Medial and lateral branches of the median nerve. The medial branch continues below the carpus as the medial volar metacarpal nerve. The lateral branch is joined by the deep branch of the ulnar (8a) to form the lateral volar metacarpal nerve.
9. Volar transverse ligament of the carpus which bridges from the medial side of the carpus to the accessory carpal bone to form the carpal canal through which the tendons of the superficial and the deep digital flexor muscles course. Note its division into superficial and deep layers.
10. Superficial volar metacarpal, or common digital artery, running behind the medial volar metacarpal vein and in front of the medial volar metacarpal nerve
11. Medial dorsal metacarpal artery
12. Anastomotic branch from the medial volar metacarpal nerve to the lateral volar metacarpal nerve
13. Superficial digital flexor tendon, in front of which can be seen a small portion of the deep digital flexor tendon (13a)
14. Distal end of the 2nd metacarpal or "splint" bone
15. Third metacarpal bone
16. Interosseous medius or suspensory ligament of the fetlock
17, 18, 19 & 20. The volar metacarpal nerve branches just above the fetlock into three branches: the dorsal digital nerve (17), the intermediate digital nerve (18) and the volar digital nerve (19). In this specimen, a small unnamed branch was dissectable going to the volar aspect of the fetlock joint (20).
21. Ergot
22. Ligament of the ergot
23. Medial proper digital artery
24. Medial proper digital vein
25. Coronary venous plexus
26. Laminar corium

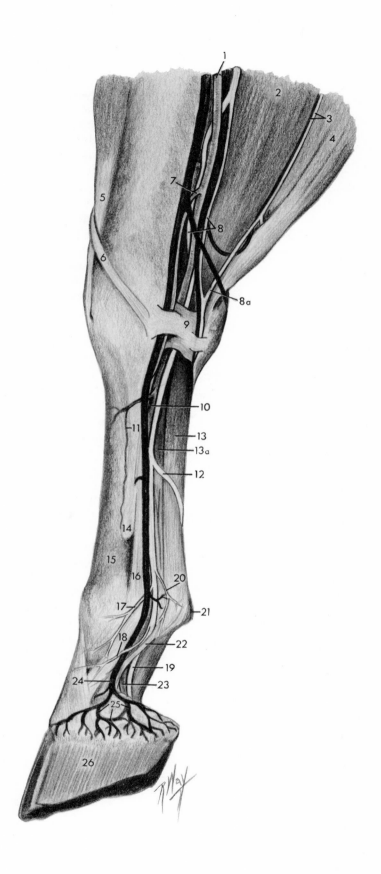

(Plate 52) 117

PLATE 53

A deeper dissection of the medial surface of the carpus. The tendon of the flexor carpi radialis muscle has been cut and the muscular portion retracted dorsally; the same procedure was followed for the flexor carpi ulnaris. The superficial layer of the volar transverse ligament of the carpus has been reflected caudally.

1. Artery of the rete carpi volare, arising from the median artery above the carpus
2. Vein of the rete carpi volare, running ventral to the artery and entering the median vein
3. The deeply situated muscular portion of the superficial and the deep digital flexors above the carpus and their tendons (3') below the carpus
4. Ulnaris lateralis, caudo-laterally
5. Superficial branch of the ulnar nerve going through an aperture in the tendon of the extensor carpi ulnaris muscle to ramify on the lateral surface of the carpus and the metacarpus
6. The point of division of the median artery, immediately above the carpus, into three terminal branches. See (7), (9) and (10).
7. The caudally running terminal branch is the lateral deep volar metacarpal artery. It can be seen anastomosing with the ulnar artery to form the supracarpal arch. The branch (7a) descending with the lateral volar metacarpal nerve (8) is still the lateral deep volar metacarpal artery.
8. Lateral branch of the median nerve inclining caudally to join with the deep branch of the ulnar nerve and form a common nerve, the lateral volar metacarpal nerve (8a)
9. Main continuation of the median artery, the superficial volar metacarpal, or common digital artery, disappearing under cover of the deep part of the volar transverse ligament of the carpus. Of the three terminal branches, this is the only one that runs through the carpal canal. Both the medial and the lateral deep volar metacarpal arteries are superficial to the deep portion of the ligament.
10. Cranial, superficial terminal branch of the median artery is the medial deep volar metacarpal artery; it runs caudal to the medial volar metacarpal vein (which is continued proximally as the cephalic vein) and then can be seen disappearing deeply just below the carpus.
11. Lateral volar metacarpal vein, ventral to the accessory carpal bone and inclining medially; it is connected by a transverse vessel with the cephalic and forms a venous loop, ventral to the arterial loop, by anastomosing with the ulnar vein. The median veins can be seen running directly upward from the lateral metacarpal vein.
12. Cut tendons of the flexor carpi radialis and the flexor carpi ulnaris
13. Medial volar metacarpal nerve, emerging below the carpus and running alongside the tendon of the deep digital flexor (caudal to the artery, in the proximal metacarpal region, and to the vein, in the distal metacarpal region)
14. Common digital artery, emerging between the vein and the nerve below the carpus and, then, disappearing again as it inclines toward the midline. In the horse, the pulse may be taken from the common digital artery in this location.
15. Medial volar metacarpal vein, ascending cranial to the nerve, in the distal metacarpal region, and cranial to the artery, in the proximal metacarpal region, and continuing as the cephalic vein
16. Anastomotic branch from the medial volar metacarpal nerve to the lateral volar metacarpal nerve, winding superficially over the caudal surface of the superficial digital flexor tendon

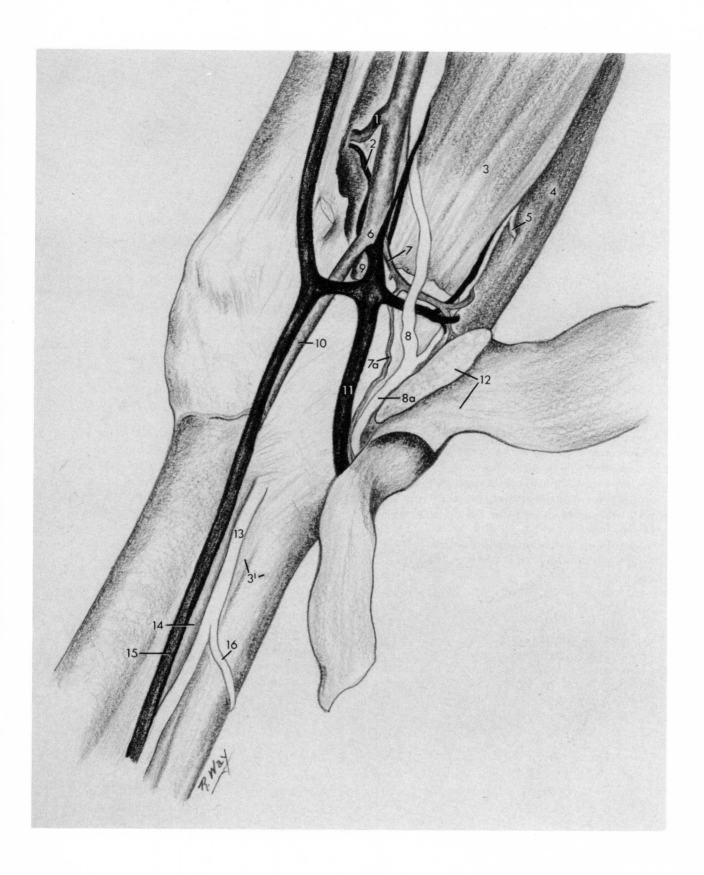

(Plate 53)   119

PLATE 54

A diagramatic representation of the volar arteries of the carpus, the metacarpus and the digit. The flexor tendons and the suspensory ligament are removed.

1. Median artery
2. Ulnar artery
3. & 4. Lateral deep volar metacarpal artery (3). It is joined by the ulnar to form the supracarpal arch (4) but continues distad in the groove between the axial side of the 4th metacarpal and the 3rd metacarpal bones.
5. Medial deep volar metacarpal artery
6. Superficial volar metacarpal, or common digital artery
7. Proximal volar arch, formed by two cross-connecting vessels, one superficial to the suspensory ligament and one deep (7'), which connects (3) and (5).
8. Dorsal metacarpal arteries, medial and lateral
9. Distal volar arch
10. Lateral proper digital artery
11. Medial proper digital artery
12. Artery of the 1st phalanx, which divides into a dorsal and a volar branch
13. Dorsal artery of the 2nd phalanx
14. Volar artery of the 2nd phalanx
15. Artery of the digital cushion
16. Dorsal artery of the 3rd phalanx
17. Terminal arch formed within the semicircular canal of the 3rd phalanx, which here has been exposed
18. Cut proximal stump of the suspensory ligament of the fetlock
19. Accessory carpal bone

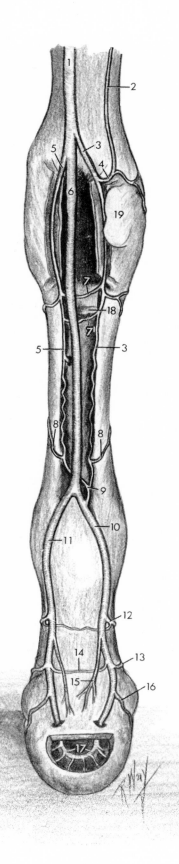

(Plate 54)   121

PLATE 55

The small arteries between the caudal surface of the third metacarpal bone and the suspensory ligament.

The ligament has been transected, its proximal half stripped away from its origin (the proximal end of the great metacarpal bone and the distal row of carpal bones) and then discarded. The distal half of the suspensory ligament remains attached to the proximal sesamoid bones. The fetlock joint capsule has been invaded, the ligaments attaching the lateral proximal sesamoid bone to the 3rd metacarpal and the 1st phalangeal bones incised, and the sesamoids, with the suspensory ligament attached, have been reflected in a hingelike manner toward the medial side.

1. Small medial interosseous muscle. Note in particular its small, thin, shiny tendon.
2. Small, medial deep volar metacarpal artery, running axial to and somewhat through the muscular head of the medial interosseous muscle
3. Smaller, lateral deep volar metacarpal artery descending on the caudal surface of the 3rd metacarpal bone and communicating with the medial artery by means of a transverse branch which arises from the medial deep volar metacarpal artery. This transverse branch may be considered a deep portion of the proximal volar arch.
4. Medial deep volar metacarpal artery giving off the nutrient artery to the great metacarpal bone and then bifurcating into tortuous terminal vessels. The medial vessel is still known as the medial deep volar metacarpal artery, the other vessel (4a) is the middle deep volar metacarpal artery.
5. Lateral deep volar metacarpal artery descending from the arch in a tortuous manner in the groove between the axial surface of the lateral small metacarpal bone (4th) and the caudal surface of the 3rd metacarpal bone.
6. The T-like arterial structure which receives the three deep volar metacarpal arteries. The medial and the middle arteries join the medial branch, the lateral artery joins the lateral branch. This confluence of arteries joining the lateral proper digital artery is known as the distal volar arch.
7. The two small collateral branches of the distal arch which descend over either side of the dorsal portion of the caudal part of the joint capsule of the fetlock joint to ramify on the craniolateral and the medial surfaces of the joint capsule.
8. Large, common digital artery (proximal portion removed)
9. Medial and the lateral proper digital arteries, arising as terminal branches from the common digital

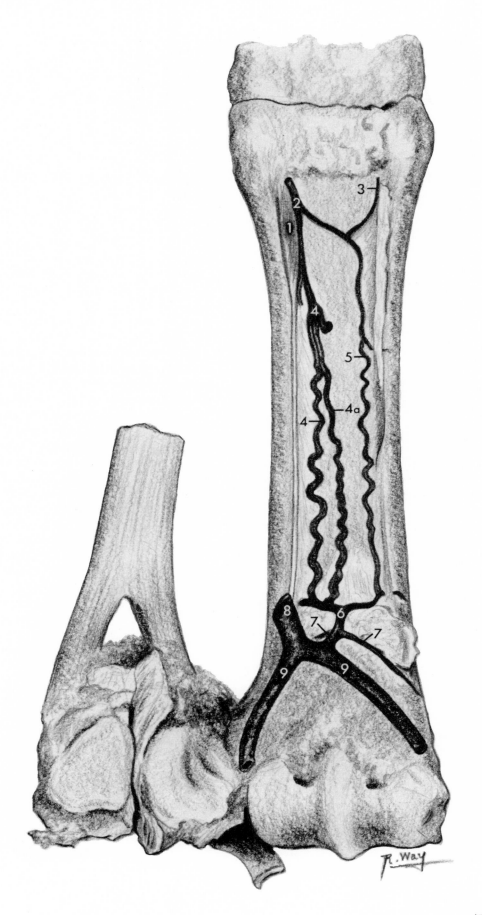

(Plate 55)   123

PLATE 56

The tendons on the dorsal side of the carpus, the metacarpus and the digit

1. Distal end of the common digital extensor muscle. Note the distal continuation of its tendon downward to the extensor process of the 3rd phalanx.

2. Distal end of the extensor carpi radialis, with its tendon extending distally to insert on the metacarpal tuberosity

3. Extensor carpi obliquus muscle, and its tendon

4. Tendon of the lateral digital extensor muscle at the point of juncture with the radial head of the common digital extensor. It then continues distally to insert on the front of the proximal end of the 1st phalanx.

5. Medial and lateral branches of the interosseous medius or suspensory ligament of the fetlock

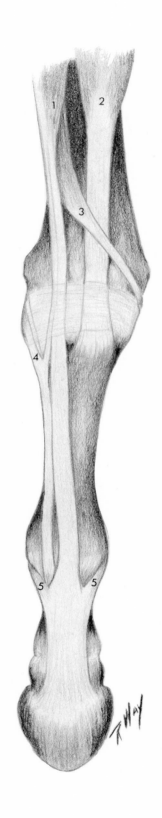

(Plate 56)   125

PLATE 57

The synovial tendon sheaths and bursae of the carpus, the metacarpus and the digit

Figure 1. Lateral view.

1. Tendon sheath of the extensor carpi radialis
2. Sheath of the common digital extensor
3. Sheath of the lateral digital extensor
4. Sheath of the long tendon of the ulnaris lateralis
5. Carpal sheath associated with both the superficial and the deep digital flexors
6. Digital sheath, which is associated with the superficial and the deep digital flexors from above the fetlock distally to the middle of the 2nd phalanx
7. Joint capsule of the fetlock joint
8. Bursa under tendon of the lateral digital extensor
9. Volar annular ligament of the fetlock
10. Proximal digital annular ligament
11. Accessory cartilage of the 3rd phalanx

Figure 2. Medial view.

1. Tendon sheath of the extensor carpi obliquus
2. Sheath of the flexor carpi radialis
3. Carpal sheath
4. Digital sheath
5. Capsule of fetlock joint
6. Accessory cartilage of the third phalanx

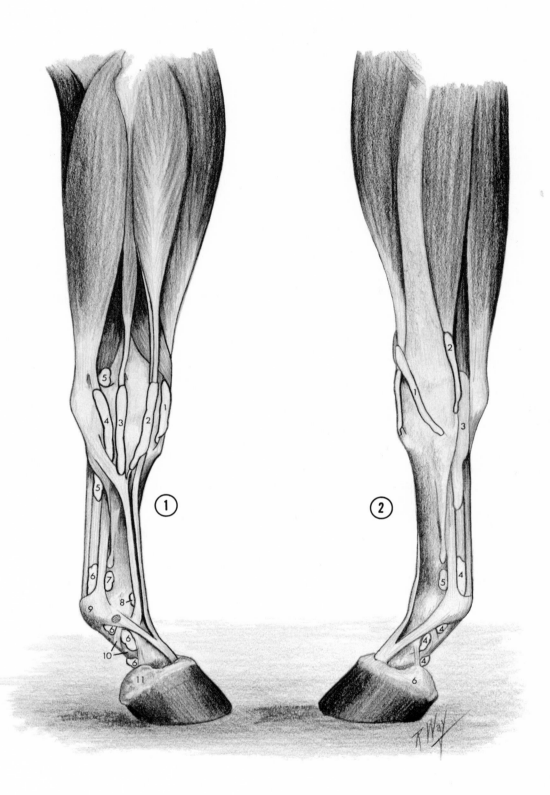

(Plate 57)   127

PLATE 58

The tendons and the ligaments of the digit

1. Abaxial branch of the suspensory ligament of the fetlock
2. Deep digital flexor tendon
3. Superficial digital flexor tendon
4. Volar annular ligament of the fetlock, which is attached to the volar surfaces of the medial and the lateral proximal sesamoid bones
5. Proximal digital annular ligament, with proximal (5a) and distal bands (5b) which are attached to the proximal and the distal collateral tubercles on the volar surface of the 1st phalanx
6. Distal digital annular ligament, which is attached to the oblique crests on either side of the distal half of the 1st phalanx. Note that the annular ligaments cover the flexor tendons and serve the purpose of fixing them in position.
7. Middle distal sesamoidean ligament, deeply situated against the bone, cranial to the deep flexor tendon
8. Central volar ligament of the pastern joint
9. Suspensory ligament of the navicular or distal sesamoid bone
10. Digital cushion, a fibro-fatty pad which lies between the frog of the hoof and the 3rd phalanx. It is an effective "shock-absorber."

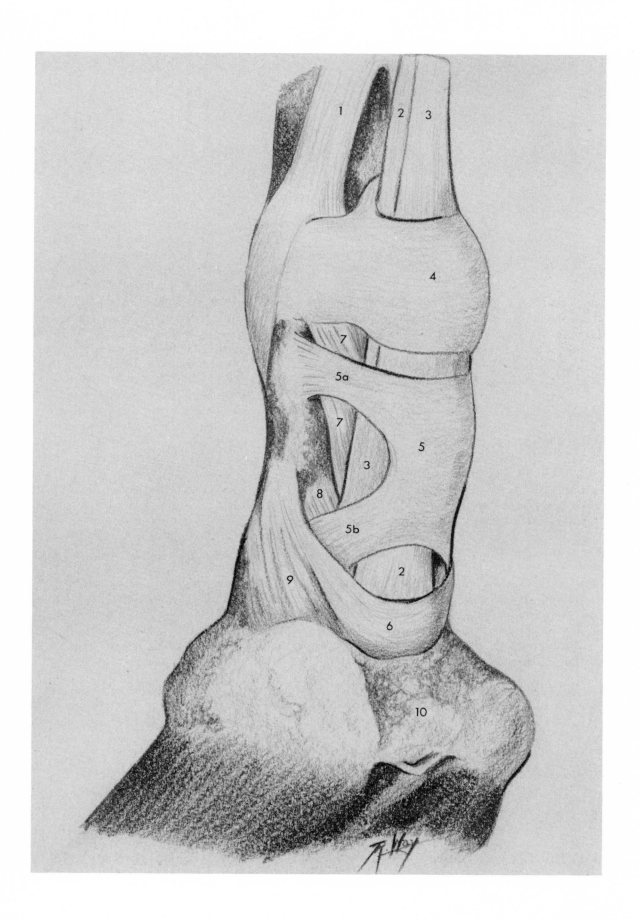

(Plate 58)   129

PLATE 59

The deep ligaments in the metacarpophalangeal region. The volar annular ligament and the proximal digital annular ligament have been incised along the midline and reflected to either side and the flexor tendons have been reflected ventrally. Refer to Plate 58 for orientation.

1. Common digital artery bifurcating into the medial and the lateral proper digital arteries above the fetlock. The distal arch can be seen entering the lateral digital artery.
2. Medial and lateral branches of the interosseous medius, or suspensory ligament of the fetlock. This may be regarded as a superior sesamoidean ligament, inasmuch as substantial portions of these branches are inserted into the proximal borders of the medial and the lateral sesamoid bones.
3. Intersesamoidean ligament, filling in the space between the two sesamoid bones
4. Superficial, or straight, distal sesamoidean ligament, arising from the intersesamoidean ligament and extending vertically to the proximal end of the 2nd phalanx

5. On either side of the superficial ligament, the strong, cordlike peripheral parts of the middle distal sesamoidean ligament, arising from the distal borders of the sesamoid bones and inserting on the triangular rough area of the volar surface of the 1st phalanx
6. The central pair of the volar ligaments of the pastern joint, arising from the volar triangular areas of the 1st phalanx and inserting on the volar side of the proximal end of the second phalanx
7. Lower limb of the proximal digital annular ligament, inserting on the distal end of the 1st phalanx between the peripheral and the central pairs of volar ligaments of the pastern joint
8. Peripheral pair of volar ligaments of the pastern joint, arising from the sides of the 1st phalanx, can be seen extending above the lower limbs of the proximal digital annular ligament. They insert on the proximal end of the 2nd phalanx and its cartilage, but this cannot be seen clearly in this illustration. These ligaments blend with the origin of the distal digital annular ligament.
9. The strong ring formed by the tendon of the superficial digital flexor muscle around the tendon of the deep digital flexor muscle (9a)
10. A second, weak loop, formed by the tendon of the superficial digital flexor muscle immediately before it bifurcates

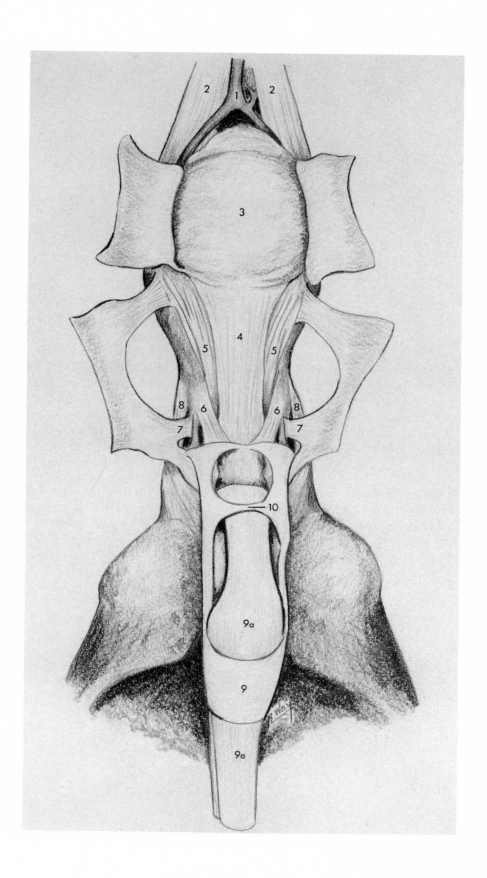

(Plate 59)   131

PLATE 60

The digital synovial sheath. The digital synovial sheath has been injected with wax to distend it abnormally in any area where it is not bound down by ligaments. In the living horse, a similar condition can occur due to an excess of synovial fluid, and the distentions are called windpuffs or windgalls.

1. & 2. The dorsal windpuff above the volar annular ligament of the fetlock. This single puff appears to be double because of the flexor tendons in the midline.

3. & 4. Windpuffs between the volar annular ligament of the fetlock and the upper branch of the proximal digital annular ligament

5. & 6. Windpuffs between the two branches of the proximal digital annular ligament

7. The ventral, median puff, visible here because the distal digital annular ligament has been removed. In the intact animal it is not evident, or only slightly so.

It must be emphasized that only under abnormal conditions, that is when the sheath contains too much synovial fluid, can these puffs be seen in the living animal.

Compare with Plates 57 and 58 for further orientation.

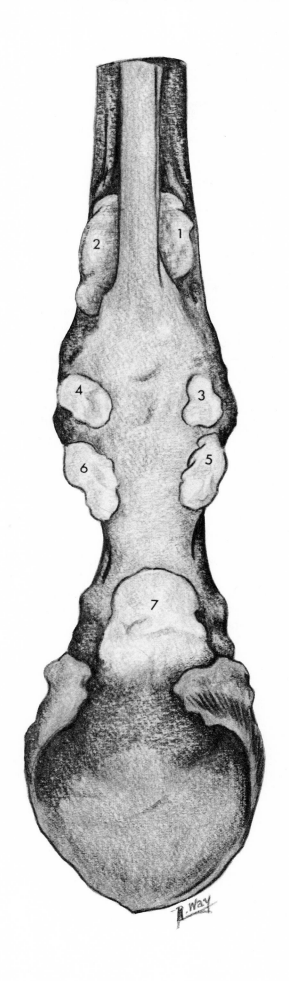

(Plate 60)   133

PLATE 61

A longitudinal median section of the distal part of the metacarpus and the digit

1. Distal end of the third metacarpal bone
2. First phalanx, or long pastern
3. Second phalanx, or short pastern
4. Third phalanx, or coffin bone
5. Distal sesamoid, or navicular bone
6. Tendon of the common digital extensor
7. Tendon of the deep digital flexor
8. Tendon of the superficial digital flexor
9. Bursa
10. Capsule of the fetlock joint
11. Cavity of the fetlock joint
12. Volar pouch of the fetlock joint capsule
13. Intersesamoidean ligament
14. Ring formed by the superficial flexor tendon which surrounds the deep flexor tendon
15. Cavity of the digital synovial sheath. Note the proximal extension above the fetlock and the distal extension to the middle of the second phalanx.
16. Ergot
17. Middle sesamoidean ligament
18. Superficial sesamoidean ligament
19. Cavity of the pastern joint
20. Cavity of the coffin joint
21. Suspensory ligament of the distal sesamoid or navicular bone
22. Navicular bursa, which lies between the navicular bone and the distal end of the deep digital flexor tendon
23. Digital cushion
24. Corium of the frog
25. Frog of the hoof
26. Corium of the sole
27. Sole of the hoof
28. Wall of the hoof
29. Laminar corium
30. Periople of the hoof
31. Coronary border of the hoof
32. Coronary corium

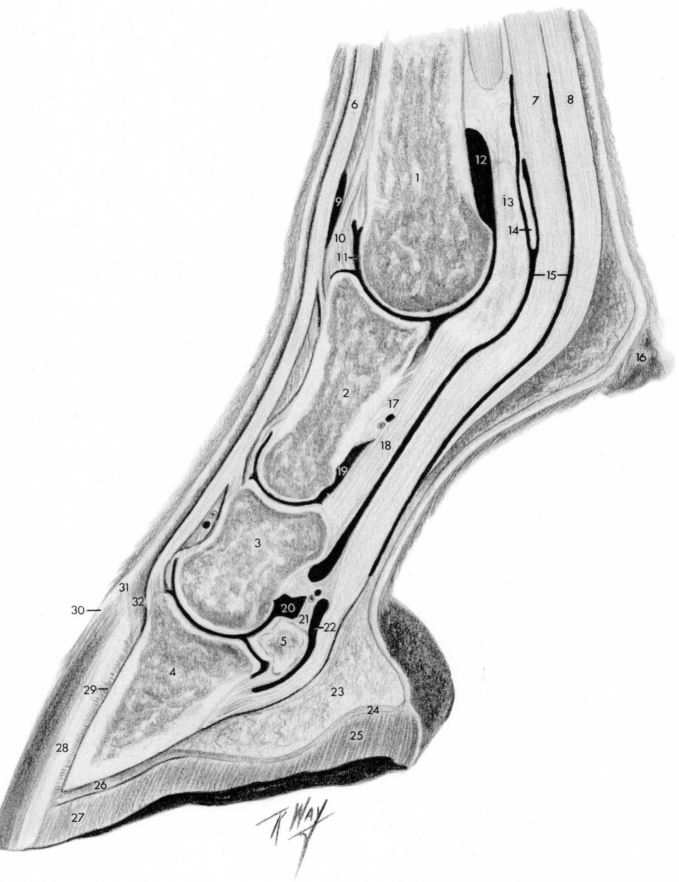

(Plate 61)   135

PLATE 62

Special postural structures of the front limb. All of the structures depicted aid in maintaining the limb in an extended position and permit the horse to sleep in the standing position without muscular fatigue.

1. The heavy tendinous tissue which covers the superficial aspect of the serratus ventralis thoracis muscle. This provides mechanical support for the trunk, since this tissue and that on the opposite side form a fibrous sling attaching the two limbs to the trunk.
2. Tendon of origin of the biceps brachii muscle
3. Tendon of insertion of the biceps brachii muscle
4. Lacertus fibrosus, a strong, fibrous band which detaches from the cranial aspect of the biceps brachii and extends downward to attach to the tendon of insertion of the extensor carpi radialis muscle. (2), (3) and (4) collectively maintain the shoulder joint in an extended position even when the extensor muscles of the joint are in the relaxed state.
5. Extensor carpi radialis muscle
6. Tendon of insertion of the superficial digital flexor muscle. Note its terminal bifurcation; one branch has been cut and deflected.
7. Radial head of the superficial digital flexor, mainly composed of fibrous tissue. Also termed the radial, or superior, check ligament.
8. Carpal, or inferior, check ligament which attaches to (9). The superior and inferior check ligaments mechanically maintain the carpus in an extended position when the antebrachial muscles are in a relaxed state.
9. Tendon of insertion of the deep digital flexor muscle
10. Suspensory ligament of the fetlock, or interosseous medius muscle
11. Tendon of insertion of the common digital extensor muscle

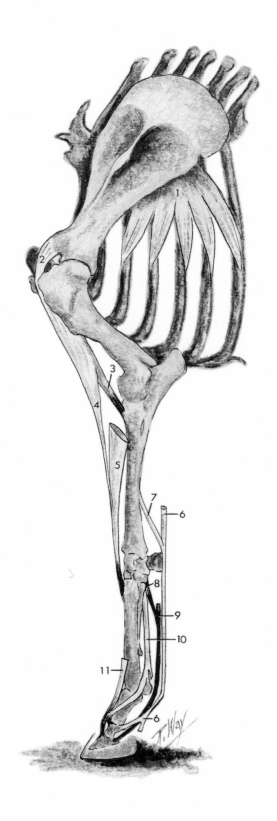

(*Plate 62*)   137

SECTION SEVEN

The Bones of the Hind Limb

PLATE 63

A cranial view of the pelvic girdle and the sacrum of a stallion

A. Sacrum
B. Pelvic surface of the left ilium
C. Left pubis
D. Left ischium

1. Spine of the 1st sacral vertebra
2. Sacral canal
3. Body of the 1st sacral vertebra
4. Articular process for articulation with the last lumbar vertebra
5. Wing of the sacrum
6. Tuber sacrale
7. Crest of the ilium
8. Tuber coxae
9. Sacrosciatic articulation
10. Shaft of the ilium
11. Greater sciatic notch
12. Sciatic spine
13. Iliopectineal line
14. Acetabulum
15. Lesser sciatic notch
16. The merged iliopectineal eminence and pubic tubercle
17. Cranial border of the pubis
18. Obturator foramen
19. Symphysis pelvis

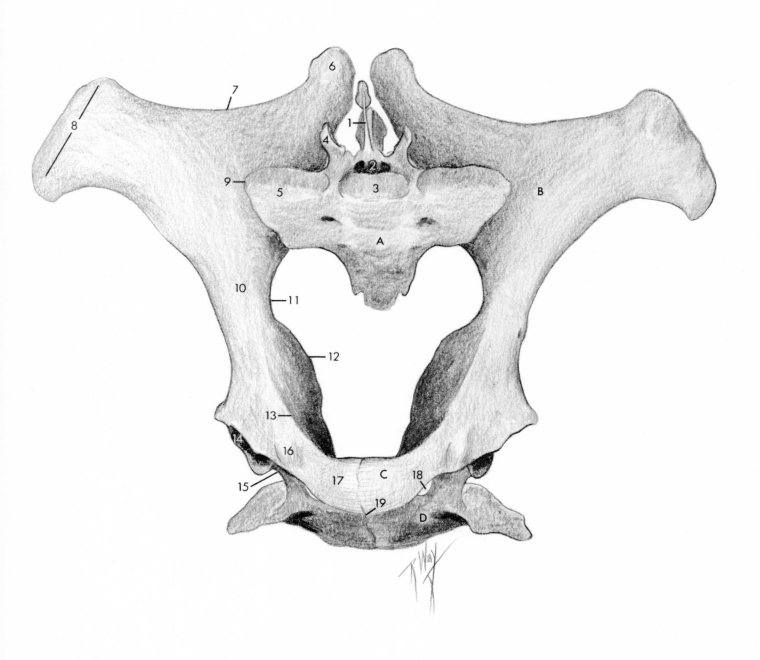

(Plate 63)   141

PLATE 64

Caudal view of the pelvic girdle and the sacrum of a stallion

A. Sacrum
B. Right ilium
C. Right pubis
D. Right ischium

1. Spine of the 5th sacral vertebra
2. Articular process for articulation with the last lumbar vertebra
3. Sacral canal
4. Body of the 5th sacral vertebra
5. Wing of the sacrum
6. Tuber sacrale
7. Gluteal line
8. Crest of the ilium
9. Gluteal surface of the ilium
10. Tuber coxae
11. Shaft of the ilium
12. Greater sciatic notch
13. Sciatic spine
14. Acetabulum
15. Lesser sciatic notch
16. Cranial border of the pubis
17. Tuber ischii
18. Ischial arch
19. Symphysis pelvis

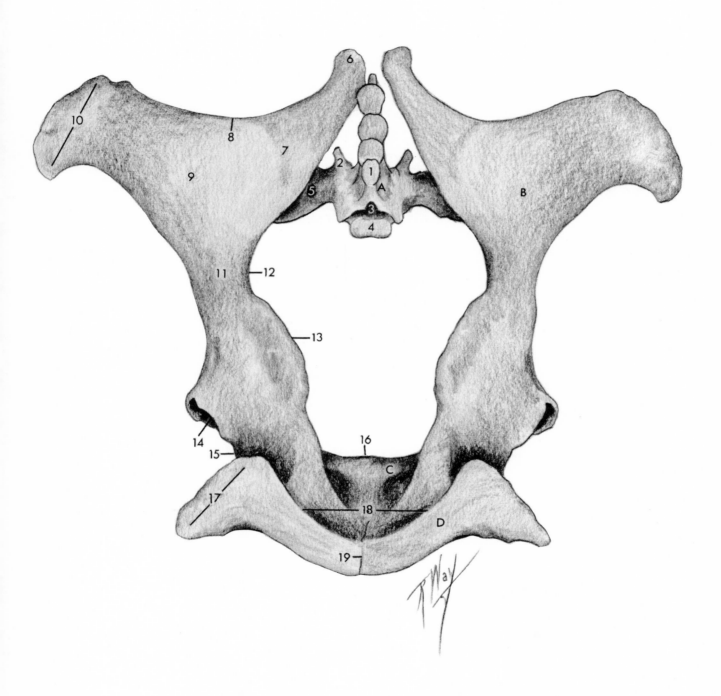

(Plate 64)   143

PLATE 65

Figure 1. The lateral aspect of the os coxae, the sacrum and associated ligaments, illustrating areas of muscular attachment.

1. Areas of origin of the tensor fascia latae
2. Area of origin of the gluteus superficialis
3. Area of origin of the gluteus medius
4. Areas of origin of the biceps femoris
5. Lateral sacro-iliac ligament
6. Area of origin of the semitendinosus
7. Area of origin of the semimembranosus
8. Sacrosciatic ligament
9. Area of origin of the biceps femoris
10. Area of origin of the gamellus
11. Area of origin of the gluteus profundus
12. Area of origin of the capsularis

13. Area of origin of the rectus femoris
14. Area of origin of the obturator externus
15. Area of origin of the adductor femoris

Figure 2. The ventral aspect of the os coxae, illustrating areas of muscular attachment.

1. Areas of origin of the rectus femoris
2. Areas of origin of the pectineus
3. Areas of origin of the obturator externus
4. Area of origin of the gracilis
5. Area of origin of the adductor femoris
6. Area of origin of the gamellus
7. Area of origin of the biceps femoris
8. Area of origin of the quadratus femoris
9. Area of origin of the semitendinosus
10. Area of origin of the semimembranosus
11. Acetabulum
12. Acetabular notch
13. Obturator foramen

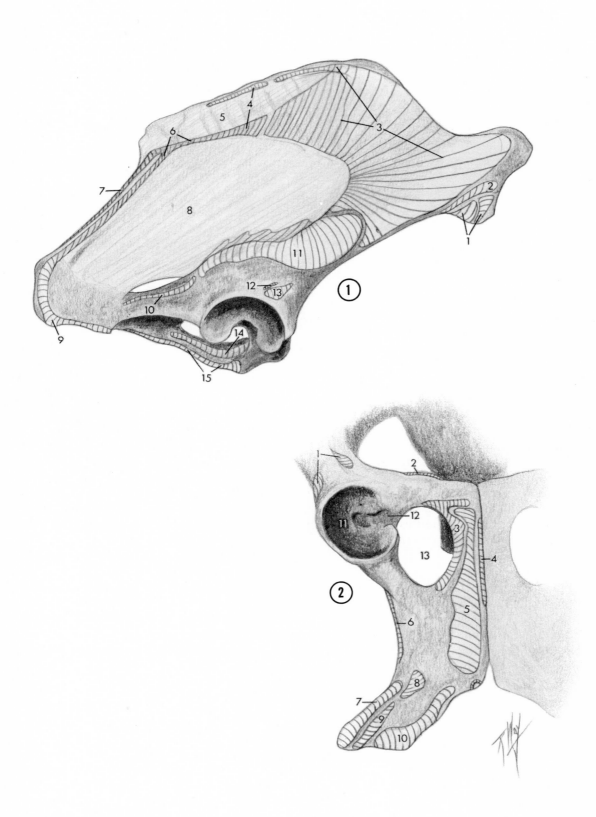

(Plate 65)   145

PLATE 66

Areas of muscular and ligamentous attachment on the femur. In all figures, corresponding areas are numbered identically.

Figure 1. Cranial view of right femur.
Figure 2. Lateral view of right femur.
Figure 3. Proximal end of right femur.
Figure 4. Caudal view of right femur.
Figure 5. Medial view of right femur.
Figure 6. Distal end of right femur.

1. Areas of insertion of the gluteus medius on the summit of the trochanter major
2. Area of insertion of the gluteus profundus on the convexity of the trochanter major
3. Area of insertion of the piriformis on the trochanteric crest. The piriformis is considered to be a portion of the gluteus medius muscle.
4. Area of insertion of the gluteus superficialis on the trochanter tertius.
5. Area of insertion of the adductor
6. Area of origin of the vastus lateralis
7. Area of origin of the lateral head of the gastrocnemius
8. Area of origin of the plantaris or superficial digital flexor from the supracondyloid fossa
9. Area of origin of the popliteus

10. Area of attachment of the lateral femoro-tibial ligament on the lateral epicondyle
11. Area of origin of the peroneus tertius and the long digital extensor from the extensor fossa
12. Area of origin of the vastus medialis
13. Area of insertion of the capsularis
14. Interval between the areas of origin of the vastus lateralis and the medialis
15. Area of insertion of the iliopsoas on the trochanter minor
16. Area of insertion of the adductor and the semimembranosus
17. Area of attachment of the medial femoro-tibial ligament on the medial epicondyle
18. Area of origin of the vastus intermedius
19. Area of origin of the medial head of the gastrocnemius from the medial supracondyloid crest
20. Area of insertion of the pectineus
21. Area of insertion of the quadratus femoris
22. Area of insertion of the biceps femoris
23. Area of insertion of the obturator externus in the lower portion of the trochanteric fossa
24. Area of insertion of the gamellus in the trochanteric fossa
25. Area of insertion of the obturator internus in the trochanteric fossa
26. Area of attachment of the caudal cruciate ligament in the intercondyloid fossa
27. Area of attachment of the femoral ligament of the lateral meniscus
28. Area of attachment of the cranial cruciate ligament

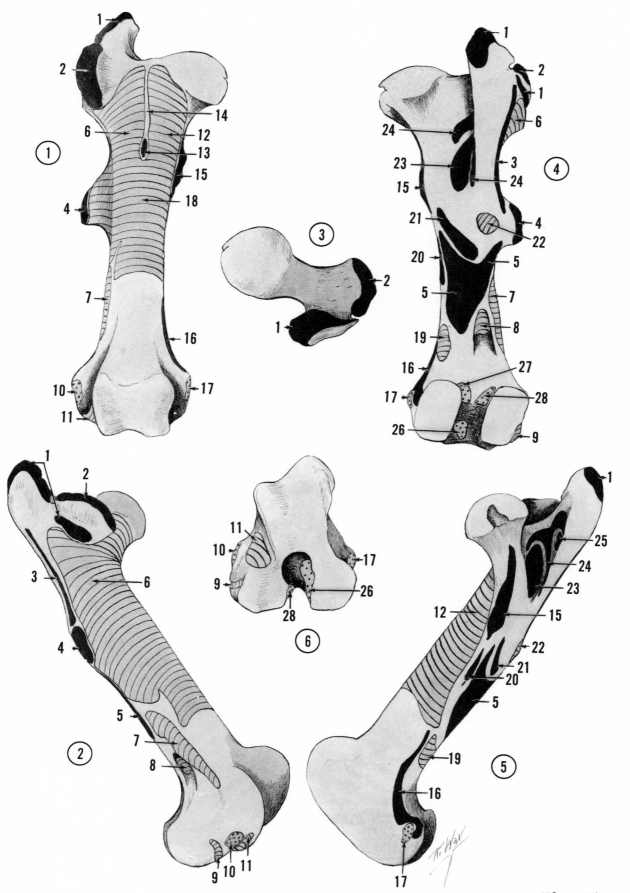

(Plate 66)   147

PLATE 67

Areas of muscular and ligamentous attachment on the tibia and fibula. In all figures corresponding areas are numbered identically.

Figure 1. Caudal view of right tibia and fibula.
Figure 2. Medial view of right tibia and fibula.
Figure 3. Lateral view of proximal end of right tibia and fibula.
Figure 4. Cranial view of proximal end of right tibia and fibula.

1. Area of origin of the caudal tibial muscle from the edge of the lateral condyle of the tibia
2. Area of origin of the long digital flexor
3. Area of attachment of the lateral femoro-tibial ligament to the proximal end of the fibula
4. Area of origin of the lateral digital extensor from the shaft of the fibula
5. Areas of origin of the flexor hallucis
6. Areas of origin of the cranial tibial muscle
7. Area of insertion of the biceps femoris on the crest of the tibia
8. Areas of attachment of the 3 patellar ligaments
9. Area of attachment of the cranial ligament of the lateral meniscus
10. Area of attachment of the cranial cruciate ligament
11. Area of attachment of the medial femoro-tibial ligament
12. Area of insertion of the gracilis
13. Area of insertion of the semitendinosus
14. Area of attachment of the cranial ligament of the medial meniscus
15. Area of attachment of the medial femoro-tibial ligament
16. Area of insertion of the popliteus
17. Area of attachment of the caudal ligament of the medial meniscus
18. Area of attachment of the cranial ligament of the medial meniscus
19. Area of attachment of caudal cruciate ligament

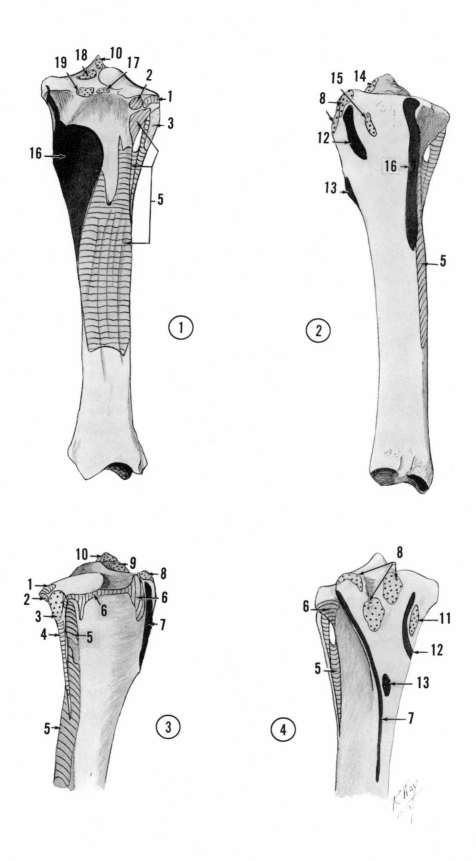

(Plate 67)   149

PLATE 68

Left tarsus (commonly referred to as the hock) and proximal end of the metatarsus. In all figures corresponding areas are numbered identically.

Figure 1. Cranial view.
Figure 2. Lateral view.
Figure 3. Caudal or plantar view.
Figure 4. Medial view.

1. Tuber calcis, or "point" of the hock
2. Body of the fibular tarsal bone
3. Medial process of the fibular tarsal bone, termed the sustentacum tali
4. Tibial tarsal bone
5. Trochlea of the tibial tarsal bone
6. Vascular canal of the tarsus
7. Central tarsal bone
8. The fused 1st and 2nd tarsal bones
9. The 3rd tarsal bone
10. The 4th tarsal bone
11. Proximal end of the 2nd metatarsal bone
12. Proximal end of the 3rd metatarsal or cannon bone
13. Proximal end of the 4th metatarsal bone

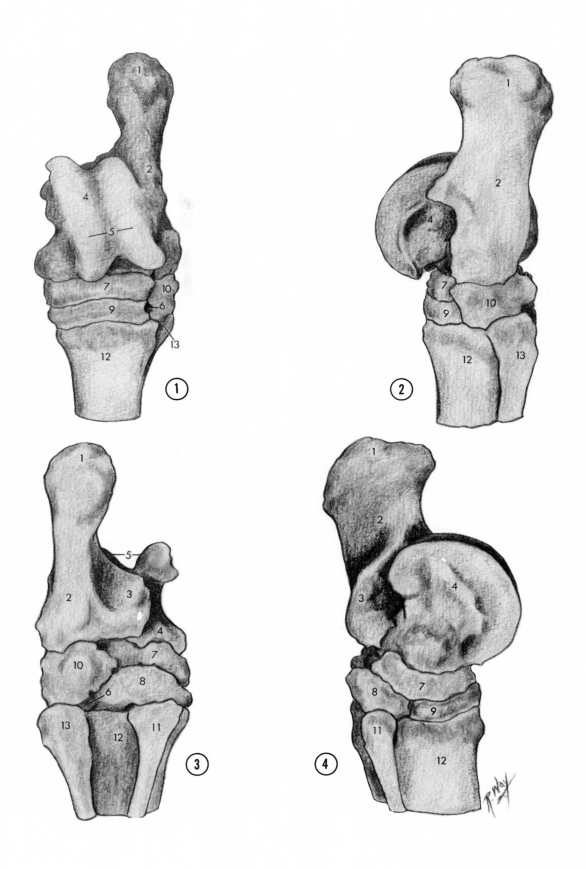

(Plate 68)   151

PLATE 69

Areas of muscular and ligamentous attachment on the bones of the right tarsus and the proximal end of the metatarsus. In all figures corresponding areas are numbered identically.

Figure 1. Lateral view.
Figure 2. Cranial view.
Figure 3. Medial view.
Figure 4. Caudal view.

1. Area of insertion of the gastrocnemius muscle
2. Area of insertion of the superficial digital flexor, the biceps femoris and the semitendinosus muscles
3. Body of the fibular tarsal bone
4. Tibial tarsal bone
5. Area of insertion of the peroneus tertius muscle
6. Fourth tarsal bone
7. Fourth metatarsal bone
8. The central tarsal bone
9. Third tarsal bone
10. Area of insertion of the peroneus tertius and tibialis cranialis muscles
11. Third metatarsal bone
12. Areas of insertion of the peroneus tertius muscle
13. The sustentaculum tali
14. Area of insertion of the tibialis cranialis muscle
15. Fused 1st and 2nd tarsal bones
16. Second metatarsal bone
17. Area of origin of the tarsal head of the deep digital flexor (the check ligament)
18. Area of origin of the interosseous medius muscle (suspensory ligament of the fetlock)

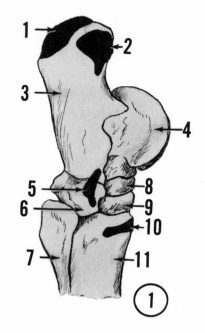

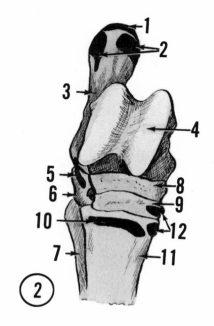

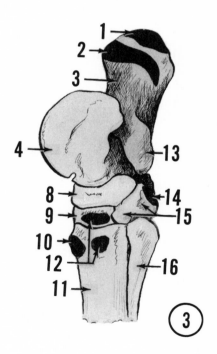

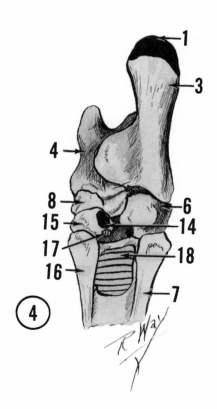

(Plate 69)   153

PLATE 70

A lateral view of the stifle joint

A. Distal end of the femur
B. Lateral and medial (B') ridges of the femoral trochlea
C. Patella
D. Lateral femoral condyle

E. Lateral tibial condyle
F. Fibula
1. Middle patellar ligament
2. Lateral patellar ligament
3. Medial patellar ligament
4. Lateral femoropatellar ligament
5. Common tendon of origin of the long digital extensor and peroneus tertius muscles
6. Cranial ligament of the lateral meniscus
7. Lateral meniscus
8. Lateral femorotibial ligament

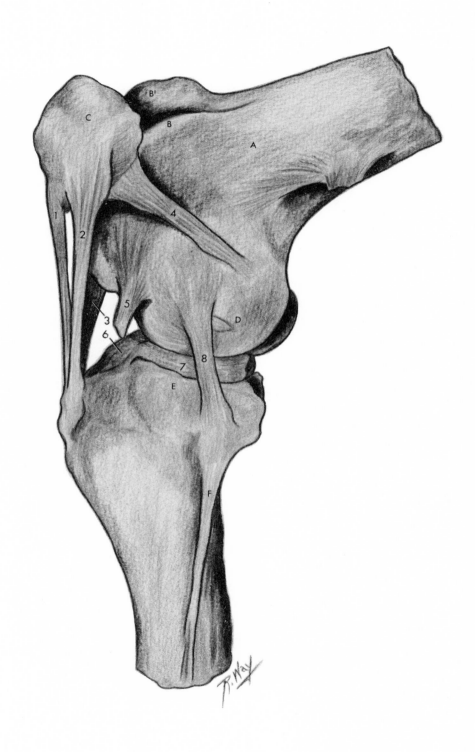

(Plate 70)   155

PLATE 71

A caudal view of the stifle joint

A. Distal end of the femur
B. Lateral and medial (B') femoral condyles
C. Lateral and medial (C') tibial condyles
D. Fibula

1. Tendon of origin of the lateral head of the gastrocnemius muscle
2. Lateral femoral-tibial ligament
3. Lateral meniscus
4. Femoral ligament of the lateral meniscus
5. Caudal ligament of the lateral meniscus
6. Lateral cruciate ligament
7. Medial cruciate ligament
8. Medial meniscus
9. Medial femoro-tibial ligament

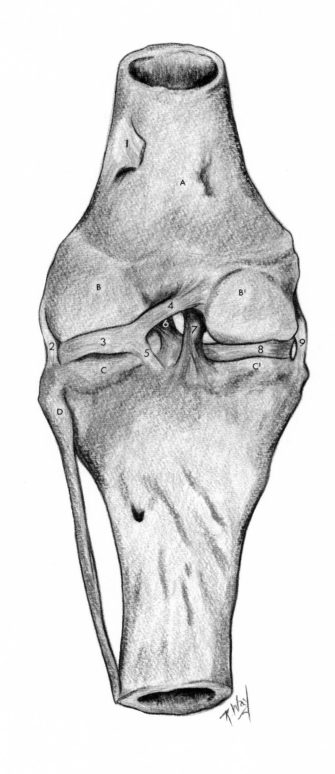

(Plate 71) 157

PLATE 72

A cranial view of the stifle joint

A. Patella
B. Medial and lateral (B') femoral condyles
C. Medial and lateral (C') tibial condyles
D. Tibial tuberosity

E. Fibula
1. Medial patellar ligament
2. Middle patellar ligament
3. Lateral patellar ligament
4. Medial femoro-tibial ligament
5. Medial meniscus
6. Common tendon of origin of the long digital extensor and the peroneus tertius muscles
7. Lateral meniscus
8. Lateral femoro-tibial ligament

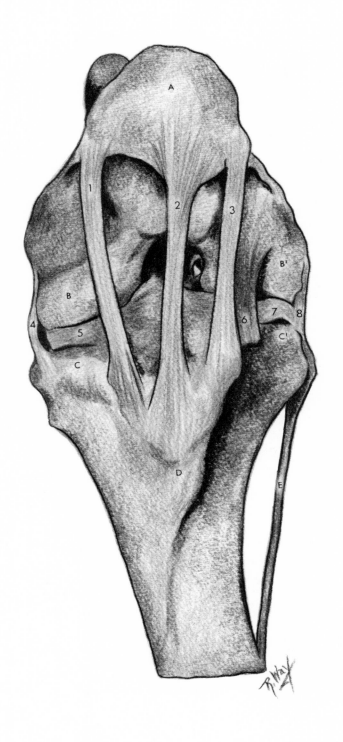

(Plate 72)   159

SECTION EIGHT

The Hind Limb

PLATE 73

The superficial muscles on the lateral aspect of the hip and the thigh and the muscles of the tail

1. Tensor fasciae latae muscle, which originates from the tuber coxae. It inserts on the fascia latae, which in turn attaches to the lateral patellar ligament and the crest of the tibia.
2. Gluteus medius muscle. This is a powerful extensor of the hip joint. It arises from the gluteal surface and the tubera of the ilium and from the dorsal and the lateral sacroiliac ligaments. Its insertion is on the trochanter major, the crest below the trochanter and the lateral aspect of the trochanteric ridge of the femur.
3. Gluteus superficialis muscle. It arises cranially from the tuber coxae and dorsally and caudally from the gluteal fascia which covers the gluteus medius and has here been removed. The insertion is to the 3rd trochanter of the femur.

4. Biceps femoris muscle, which arises from the dorsal and the lateral sacro-iliac ligaments, the gluteal and the coccygeal fascia and the tuber ischii. It inserts on the caudal surface of the femur behind the 3rd trochanter, the lateral surface of the patella and the lateral patellar ligament, the tibial crest, the crural fascia and the tuber calcis. Note that, below, the muscle has three divisions.
5. Semitendinosus muscle, which arises from the first two coccygeal vertebrae and from the ventral surface of the tuber ischii. Its insertion is on the tibial crest, the crural fascia and the tuber calcis.
6. Caudal border of the semimembranosus
7. Coccygeus muscle, a depressor of the tail
8. Lateral part of the sacro-coccygeus ventralis muscle
9. Intertransversales caudae muscles
10. Sacro-coccygeus lateralis muscle
11. Sacro-coccygeus dorsalis muscle

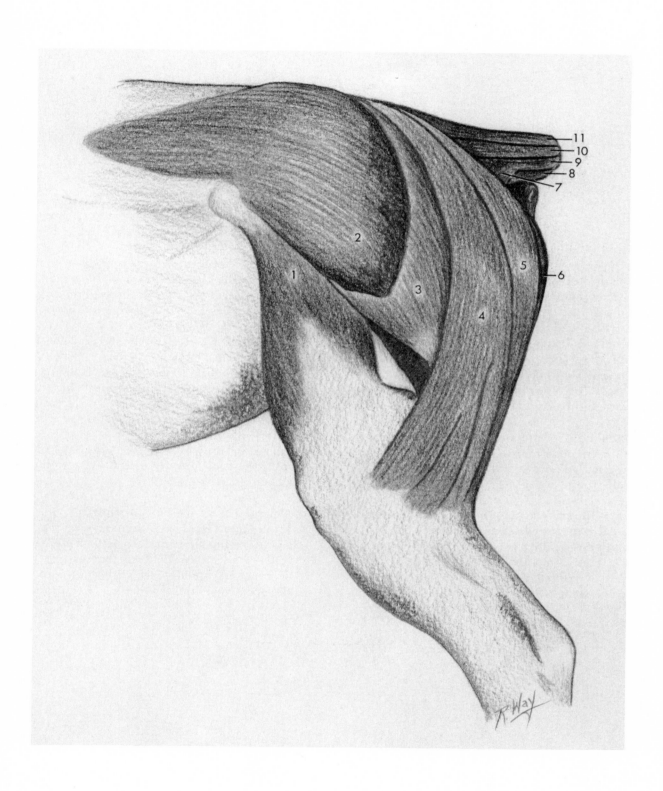

(Plate 73)   163

PLATE 74

The deep gluteal region and the sacral portion of the lumbosacral plexus

To prepare this specimen, the gluteal fascia and the superficial and the middle gluteal muscles have been removed, leaving only small portions of their insertions. The biceps femoris and the semitendinosus muscle have been dissected from their origins at the sacroiliac ligament and allowed to hang downward and backward.

1. Caudal belly of the tensor fasciae latae muscle, arising from a strong septum which is attached to the lateral border of the ilium. Note, also, the small stump of muscle, just behind the tensor fasciae latae and also arising from this septum. This is the cut proximal belly of the superficial gluteal muscle. Observe the nerve (below the stump) descending to supply the tensor fasciae latae. This a branch of the cranial gluteal nerve.
2. Accessory gluteal muscle, arising from the wing and the shaft of the ilium, lateral to the gluteal line, and its long tendon of insertion riding over the convexity of the great trochanter of the femur to insert below on the crest of the great trochanter
3. Portion of the fleshy vastus lateralis muscle arising from the lateral surface of the femur
4. Cut tendon of insertion of the superficial gluteal muscle, attached to the trochanter tertius of the femur
5. Summit of the great trochanter and the lateral surface of the trochanteric ridge on which the muscular fibers of the middle gluteal muscle (gluteus medius) can be seen inserting
6. Portion of the deep gluteal muscle (gluteus profundus), deep to the middle and the accessory gluteal muscles
7. Dorsal sacroiliac ligament, cordlike, running from the tuber sacrale of the ilium to the coccygeal dorsal spines
8. Lateral sacroiliac ligament, triangular in shape, attaching to the medial border of the wing of the ilium cranially. It is continuous with the dorsal sacroiliac ligament dorsally and caudally. Ventrally, it is attached to the lateral part of the sacrum and caudally is directly continuous with the coccygeal fascia, which has been removed.

9. Muscles of the tail. The midline, which can be seen dorsally, is the division between the left and the right dorsal sacrococcygeus muscles. Immediately under the dorsal muscle is the long, narrow lateral sacrococcygeus muscle; below this is the small, intertransversales caudae muscle and, finally, the ventral sacrococcygeus muscle. Note the small crescentic muscle, lateral to the ventral sacrococcygeal muscle, inserting on and between the fibers of the intertransversales and thereby onto the transverse processes of the coccygeal vertebrae. This is the coccygeus muscle.

10. Anus, below the tail

11. Several cut stumps of the cranial gluteal artery, which can be seen emerging through the greater sciatic foramen. These severed branches were supplying the middle gluteal muscle.

12. Large, flat band of nervous tissue which represents the caudal part of the lumbosacral plexus. The cut stump of the cranial gluteal nerve can be seen just behind the cranial gluteal artery. Another portion of this nerve can be seen disappearing under cover of the accessory gluteal muscle to run between that muscle and the deep gluteal muscle, coursing laterally to reach the tensor fasciae latae. As was mentioned previously, the distal portion can be seen entering the medial surface of the latter muscle. Observe the wide band which is subdivided into two portions running downward and backward over the dorsal portion of the deep gluteal muscle, then behind the hip joint to descend almost vertically behind the femur. The cranial portion is the common peroneal nerve (12a); the caudal portion is the sciatic nerve (12b). Note the large muscular branch of the sciatic behind the hip joint which supplies the biceps femoris and the semitendinosus muscles.

Observe the long, thin nerve above the sciatic. This is the ventral branch of the caudal gluteal nerve (12c). Note that part of it pierces the fibrous wall of the pelvic cavity and the remainder continues downward and backward as the caudal cutaneous nerve of the thigh (12d). The latter runs through the fibers of origin of the biceps femoris from the tuber ischii (stump remaining) to emerge between the biceps and the semitendinosus muscles below the tuber ischii and ramify on the caudal thigh region.

Above the ventral branch of the caudal gluteal nerve, note the dorsal branch (12e) whose

(Plate 74)   165

branches supply the middle and the superficial gluteal, the biceps femoris and the semitendinosus muscles.

13. Caudal gluteal artery and vein immediately dorsal to the dorsal branch of the caudal gluteal nerve. Observe the small ischiatic lymph nodes on the course of this artery.

14. Small portion of the internal pudendal artery and vein (just above the cut stump of the gluteus medius muscle) emerging from the pelvic cavity and shortly re-entering it.

15. Immediately behind and below the internal pudendal artery, observe the internal obturator muscle emerging from the pelvic cavity by squeezing through the lesser sciatic foramen.

16. Strong, fibrous wall medial to the nerves. This is the sacrosciatic ligament and is directly continuous above with the lateral sacroiliac ligament, where they are attached in common to the lateral part of the sacrum and the transverse processes of the 1st and the 2nd coccygeal vertebrae. Its ventral border is attached to the dorsal ischiatic spine and the tuber ischii, and, between these, it bridges over the lateral border of the ischium, forming the lesser sciatic foramen. The caudal border is fused with the vertebral origin of the semimembranosus muscle which can be easily seen. The cranial border cannot be domonstrated because of the large nerves and the cranial gluteal artery emerging through the greater sciatic foramen here.

17. Just behind the trochanter tertius, note the attachment of the biceps femoris muscle to the caudal surface of the femur.

18. Medial to the attachment of the biceps to the femur, observe the deep femoral artery and vein emerging from a cleft between the quadratus femoris muscle dorsally and the adductor muscle ventrally, to enter the substance of the biceps femoris muscle.

19. Large vein, the caudal femoral, ascending medial to the muscular branch of the sciatic nerve to disappear under the ischium, where it joins the obturator vein

20. Deep arteries and veins entering the semimembranosus and the semitendinosus muscles. These are branches of the obturator artery and vein.

21. Semitendinosus muscle's origin from the ischium. The dorsal part of the muscle has been allowed to hang downward and backward.

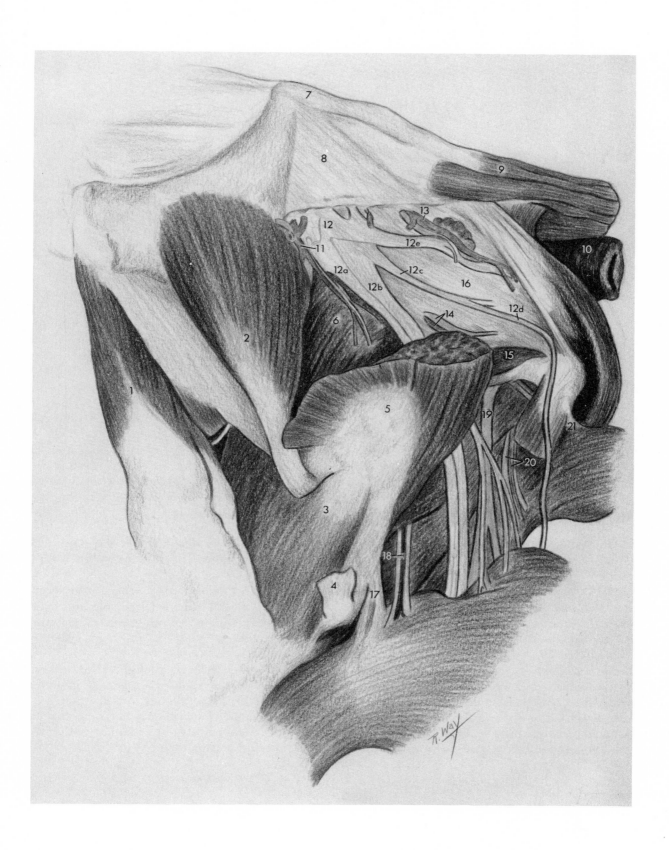

(Plate 74)   167

PLATE 75

The caudal part of the sacral plexus, the pelvic diaphragm and the muscles of the tail

The lateral sacroiliac ligament has been dissected from the dorsal sacroiliac ligament, the medial border of the wing of the ilium and the lateral part of the sacrum. The latter procedure, of course, freed the ventrally continuous sacrosciatic ligament, and both ligaments have been allowed to hang ventrolaterally. This procedure exposes the ventral rami of the caudal sacral nerves, the muscles of the tail and the muscles which close the pelvic cavity and with their fellows form sort of a pelvic diaphragm.

1. Dorsal sacro-iliac ligament, attaching to the summits of the sacral and the first few coccygeal vertebrae
2. Paired sacrococcygeus dorsalis muscles on either side of the midline
3. Lateral sacrococcygeus muscle, arising from the lateral surface of the sacrum and the coccygeal vertebrae
4. Muscular fibers which seem to be a forward continuation of the lateral sacrococcygeus muscle form the multifidus dorsi muscle
5. Ventral ramus of the 2nd sacral nerve emerging from the ventral surface of the sacrum and then disappearing lateral to the sacrosciatic ligament
6. Lateral sacral artery and its large terminal branch, the caudal gluteal artery, which pierces the sacrosciatic ligament, and its other small terminal branch, the lateral coccygeal artery, which disappears between the intertransversales caudae and ventral sacrococcygeus muscles and supplies the tail
7. Ventral rami of the 3rd and the 4th sacral nerves and an anastomotic branch connecting them immediately under the lateral coccygeal artery

Two parallel, named nerves descend medial to the sacrosciatic ligament. The cranial nerve is the pudendal nerve and the caudal one is the caudal hemorrhoidal nerve.

8. Pudendal nerve descending lateral to both muscles which form the left portion of the pelvic diaphragm. Note that it detaches a branch which receives a branch from the caudal gluteal nerve and the combined nerve courses caudally to ramify around the anus and the perineum. Observe that the caudal gluteal nerve continues ventrally, imbedded in the sacrosciatic ligament. This nerve descends to supply the ischiocavernosus muscle. The major portion of the pudendal nerve continues ventrally, passes over the lateral surface of the internal pudendal artery and then disappears from sight ventral to the artery.
9. Internal pudendal artery, bifurcating into a small, ascending perineal artery, and its direct continuation the artery of the bulb (in the male)
10. Coccygeus muscle, arising from the dorsal ischiatic spine and the surrounding portion of sacrosciatic ligament and inserting on the transverse processes of the coccygeal vertebrae and the coccygeal fascia
11. Retractor ani muscle, ventral to (10) and forming with it one side of the pelvic diaphragm. Its insertion is directly into the sphincter muscle fibers of the anus.
12. Caudal hemorrhoidal nerve, disappearing medial to the coccygeus muscle and lateral to the retractor ani and ramifying with a branch of the pudendal nerve in the anal and perineal region
13. Anal lymph nodes, situated on the dorsolateral surface of the retractor ani muscle immediately ventral to the coccygeus muscle
14. Ventral sacrococcygeus muscle, medial to the coccygeus muscle and medial to the ventral rami of the sacral nerves

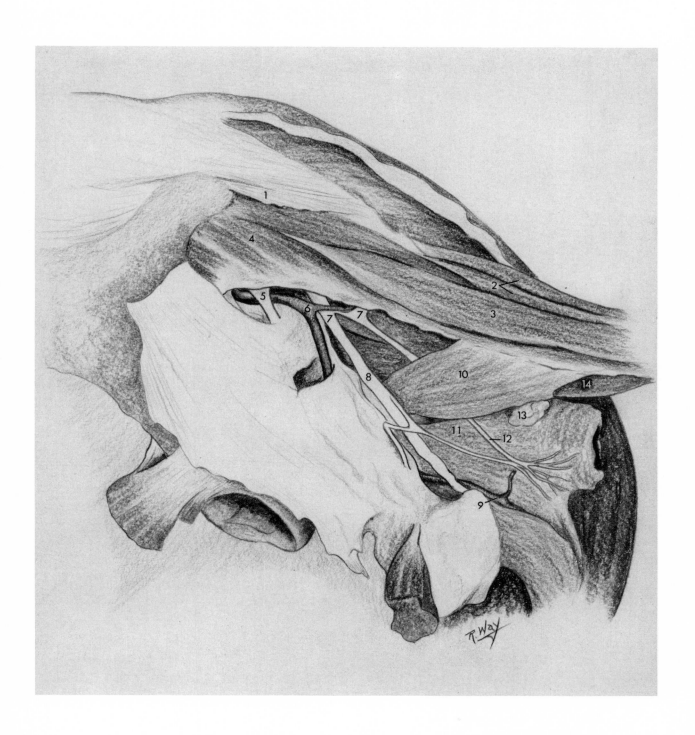

(Plate 75) 169

PLATE 76

A deep dissection of the lateral aspect of the pelvis. The gluteal muscles, the biceps femoris and the coccygeal origin of the semitendinosus muscle have been removed.

1. Ilium, gluteal surface
2. Lateral sacroiliac ligament
3. Sacrosciatic ligament
4. Iliolumbar artery
5. Branch of the cranial gluteal nerve to the tensor fasciae latae muscle
6. Branches of the iliaco-femoral artery
7. Cranial gluteal artery and nerve
8. Sciatic nerve
9. Dorsal and ventral branches of the caudal gluteal nerve
10. Caudal gluteal artery
11. Ischiatic lymph node
12. Pudendal nerve
13. Internal pudendal artery
14. Caudal cutaneous femoral nerve
15. Muscular branch of sciatic nerve
16. Tibial nerve
17. Peroneal nerve
18. Proximal end of the gluteus medius muscle
19. Proximal end of the tensor fasciae latae muscle
20. Rectus femoris muscle
21. Trochanteric bursa, which has been cut open when the gluteus accessorius tendon was reflected distally
22. Tendon of insertion of the gluteus medius muscle
23. Vastus lateralis muscle
24. Tendon of insertion of the obturator internus muscle
25. Gamellus muscle
26. Obturator externus muscle
27. Quadratus femoris muscle
28. Terminal branches of the obturator artery
29. Semitendinosus muscle
30. Semimembranosus muscle

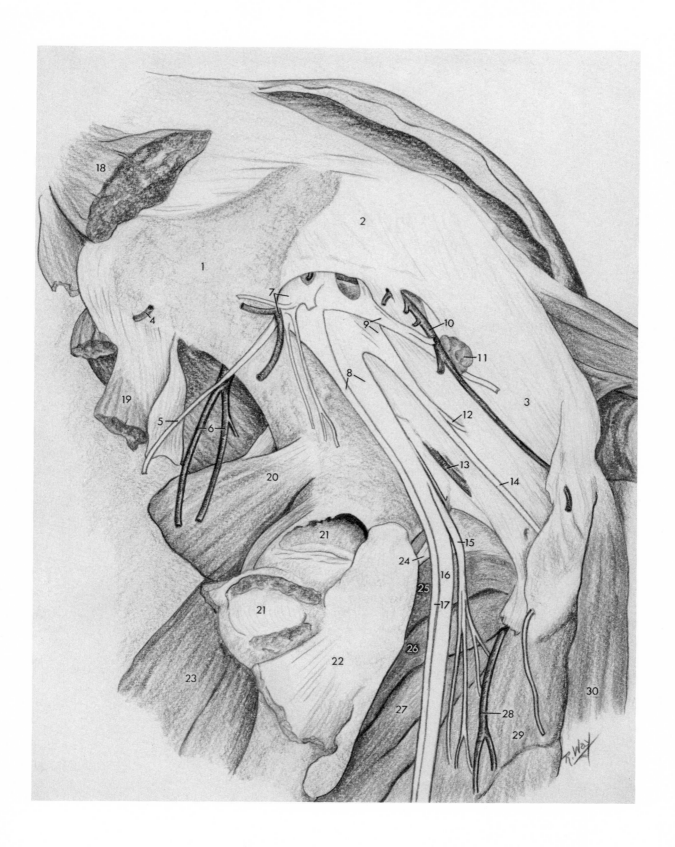

(Plate 76)   171

PLATE 77

A dissection of the pelvis illustrating in detail the lumbosacral nerve plexus. The pelvic veins have been removed and the arteries detached and reflected downward.

The lumbosacral plexus is formed chiefly from the union of the ventral branches of the last three lumbar and first two sacral spinal nerves. The nerves which innervate the pelvic limb are derived from the plexus.

1, 2 & 3. Ventral branches of the 4th, the 5th and the 6th lumbar nerves
4 & 5. Ventral branches of the 1st and the 2nd sacral nerves, which emerge from the 1st and the 2nd ventral sacral foramina
6 & 7. The 5th and 6th lumbar vertebrae
8. Sacrum
9. Sympathetic trunk. Note the communicating rami to the lumbar and sacral nerves.
10. Femoral nerve
11. Obturator nerve
12. Cranial gluteal nerve
13. Sciatic nerve
14. Caudal gluteal nerve, which promptly divides into dorsal and ventral branches
15. Caudal cutaneous femoral nerve, a branch of the caudal gluteal
16 & 17. The 3rd and the 4th sacral nerves, ventral branches
18. Pudendal nerve
19. Caudal hemorrhoidal nerve
20. Pelvic nerves. These continue downward to a flap of detached pelvic fascia (20a) within which they branch to form a pelvic plexus.
21. The stump of the deep circumflex iliac artery
22. The external iliac
23. Internal iliac or hypogastric artery
24. Internal pudendal artery
25. Stump of the umbilical artery
26. Stump of the lateral sacral artery. A portion of this vessel had to be removed to uncover the sacral nerves. Its terminal end (26') may be seen caudal to (16) where it divides into caudal gluteal (26a) and lateral sacral branches (26b).
27. Iliacofemoral artery
28. Obturator artery
29. Cranial gluteal artery
30. Psoas major muscle
31. Psoas minor muscle
32. Iliacus muscle
33. Tensor fasciae latae muscle
34. Rectus femoris muscle
35. Vastus medialis muscle
36. Prepubic tendon
37. Pubis, cut sagittally at the symphysis pelvis

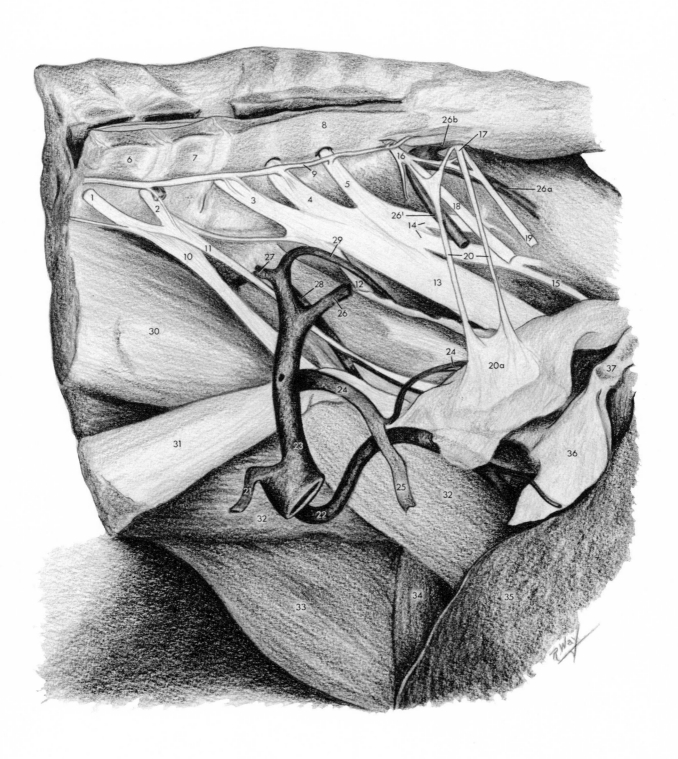

(Plate 77)   173

PLATE 78

The suspensory apparatus of the anus

The procedure followed to prepare this deep dissection was to incise the coccygeus and the retractor ani muscles at their insertions and reflect them laterally. Then the outer, connective tissue coat of the rectum was incised and also reflected laterally which exposed the smooth muscle coat of the rectum. The fusiform ventral sacrococcygeus muscle was incised and its proximal lateral portion reflected laterally.

1. Major portion of the caudal hemorrhoidal nerve entering the medial surface of the coccygeus muscle (1a), while a smaller branch descends to reach the lateral surface of the retractor ani muscle (1b) and the peroneal region
2. Heavy white connective tissue coat of the rectum
3. Smaller, inner portion of the ventral sacrococcygeus muscle, the ventral sacrococcygeus medialis, is clearly exposed when the larger, ventral sacrococcygeus lateralis muscle (3a) is transected and its cranial portion allowed to hang laterally.
4. Muscular coat of the rectum, sweeping up on either side of the midline to insert onto the bodies of the 4th and the 5th coccygeal vertebrae. This is the rectococcygeus muscle. Note the very small middle coccygeal artery (4a) emerging through the substance of the rectococcygeus and descending along the midline of the ventral surface of the tail.
5. Suspensory ligament of the anus, a band of smooth muscle, arising from the first coccygeal vertebra and passing downward on either side of the anus. Note that it is continued ventrally as the retractor penis muscle (5a).
6. External sphincter muscle of the anus, surrounding the anal orifice
7. Strong, paired ischiocavernosus muscles surrounding the crura of the penis below the anus

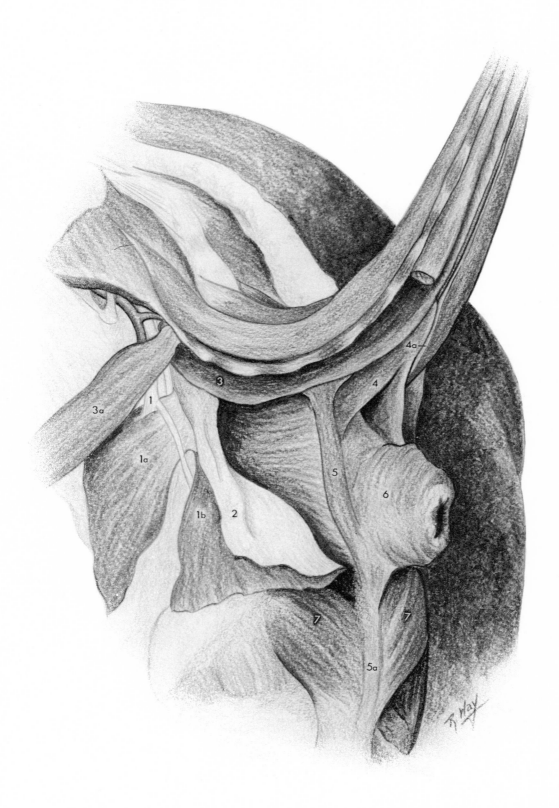

(Plate 78)   175

PLATE 79

The sublumbar muscles and the medial muscles of the femoral or thigh region

1. Caudal end of the psoas minor muscle, which originates from the bodies of the last three thoracic and the first four lumbar vertebrae and the vertebral ends of the 16th and the 17th ribs. It inserts on the psoas tubercle located on the cranial portion of the shaft of the ilium.
2. Caudal end of the psoas major muscle, which arises from the ventral surfaces of the transverse processes of the lumbar vertebrae and the last two ribs. It inserts on the trochanter minor of the femur.
3. Iliacus muscle, which arises from the ventral surface of the ilium, the ventral sacro-iliac ligament, the wing of the sacrum and the tendon of the psoas minor. It inserts on the trochanter minor of the femur by a common tendon with the psoas major. The psoas major and the iliacus are so intimately united that they are often considered to form a single muscle termed the iliopsoas muscle.
4. Sartorius muscle, which originates from the iliac fascia and the tendon of insertion of the psoas minor. Distally, it inserts on the medial patellar ligament and the tuberosity of the tibia.
5. External iliac artery
6. Common trunk which gives rise to the deep femoral artery and the prepubic artery (8). The deep femoral courses caudally to disappear beneath the pectineus muscle (11).
7. The femoral artery, which is a direct continuation of the external iliac artery
8. Prepubic artery
9. Deep inguinal lymph nodes
10. Quadriceps femoris muscle
11. Pectineus muscle
12. The gracilis muscle, which originates from the pelvic symphysis, the prepubic tendon and the accessory ligament and from the ventral surface of the pubis. It inserts on the medial patellar ligament, the medial surface of the proximal end of the tibia and the crural fascia.
13. Semitendinosus muscle
14. Saphenous vein
15. Saphenous nerve
16. Pelvic cavity, from which all visceral organs have been removed

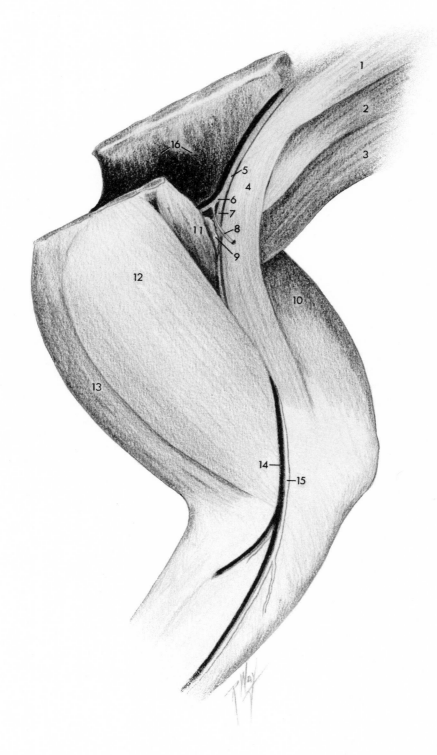

(Plate 79) 177

PLATE 80

The sublumbar and the medial muscles of the femoral region. This plate differs from the preceding one in that the gracilis and the sartorius muscles have been detached from their origin and reflected downward.

1. Psoas minor muscle
2. Psoas major muscle
3. Sartorius muscle
4. Quadriceps femoris muscle
5. Pectineus muscle
6. Adductor muscle
7. Semimembranosus muscle, which originates on the caudal border of the sacrosciatic ligament and the ventral surface of the tuber ischii. It inserts on the medial epicondyle of the femur.
8. The semitendinosus muscle, which arises from the transverse processes of the 1st and the 2nd coccygeal vertebrae and the ventral surface of the tuber ischii. It inserts on the crest of the tibia, the crural fascia and the tuber calcis.
9. Medial head of the gastrocnemius muscle
10. Reflected gracilis muscle
11. Reflected sartorius muscle

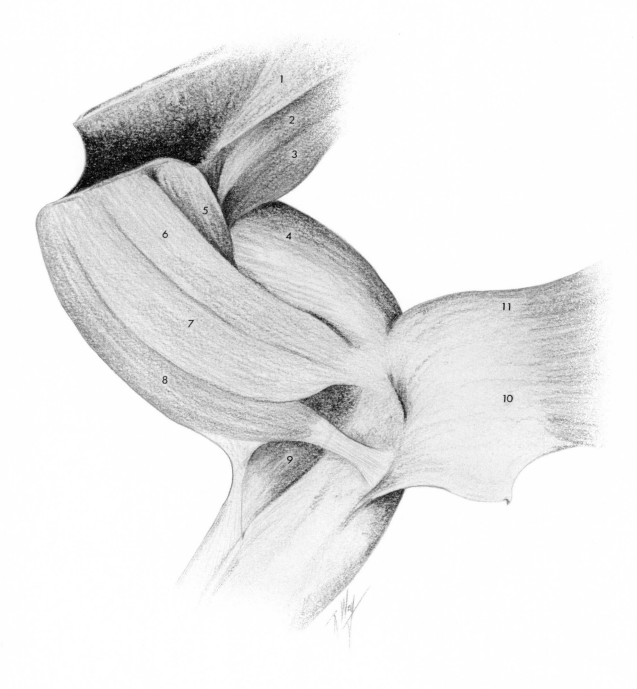

(Plate 80)   179

PLATE 81

The sublumbar and the medial muscles of the thigh. The gracilis, the semimembranosus and the sartorius muscles have been detached from their origins and reflected to the right.

1. Psoas minor muscle
2. Psoas major muscle
3. Iliacus muscle
4. External iliac artery
5. Pectineus muscle
6. Quadriceps femoris muscle
7. Femoral artery
8. Adductor muscle, which arises from the ventral surface of the pubis and the ischium and inserts on the caudal surface of the femur, the medial epicondyle of the femur and the medial ligament of the stifle joint
9. Branch of the obturator nerve which innervates the gracilis muscle. This was cut when the gracilis was reflected.
10. Semitendinosus muscle
11. Sciatic nerve
12. Branch of the sciatic nerve entering the medial or deep face of the biceps femoris muscle
13. Caudal cutaneous crural branch of the sciatic nerve
14. Tibial nerve—the direct continuation of the sciatic
15. Fibular, or peroneal, nerve
16. Terminal portion of the femoral artery. Here the artery dips between the medial and the lateral heads of the gastrocnemius muscle to be continued as the popliteal artery.
17. Reflected semimembranosus muscle
18. Reflected gracilis and sartorius muscles

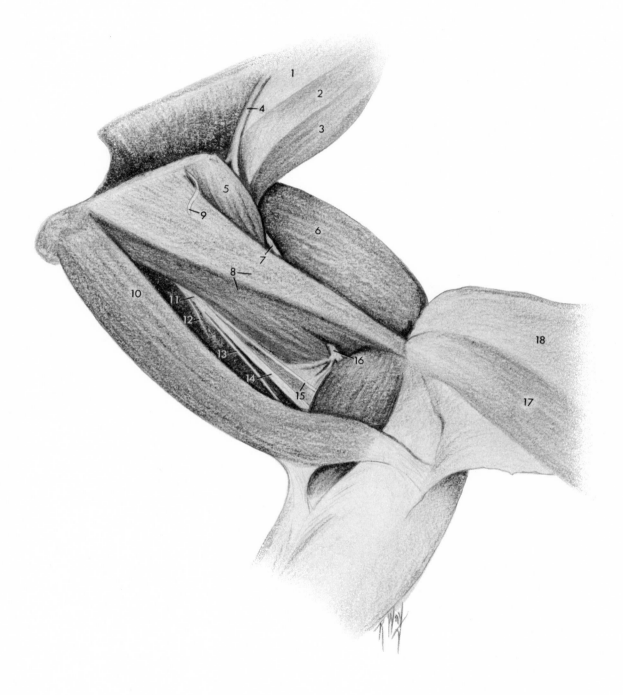

(Plate 81)   181

PLATE 82

Deep dissection of the sublumbar and the medial femoral muscles, illustrating also the principal arteries and nerves of the region

1. Psoas minor muscle
2. Psoas major muscle
3. Iliacus muscle
4. External iliac artery
5. The pectineus muscle, which arises from the prepubic tendon, the accessory ligament and the cranial border of the pubis. It inserts on the medial border of the femur.
6. Branch of the obturator nerve
7. Obturator externus muscle
8. Branches of the caudal gluteal artery and nerve to the semitendinosus muscle
9. Quadratus femoris muscle, which arises from the ventral surface of the ischium and inserts on the caudal surface of the femur near the lower portion of the trochanter minor
10. Semitendinosus muscle
11. Sciatic nerve
12. Medial or deep face of the biceps femoris muscle
13. Medial surface of the femur
14. Femoral artery
15. Quadriceps femoris muscle
16. Caudal femoral artery, with its ascending and descending branches
17. Popliteal artery
18. Medial head of the gastrocnemius muscle
19. Reflected semimembranosus muscle
20. Reflected abductor muscle
21. Reflected sartorius muscle

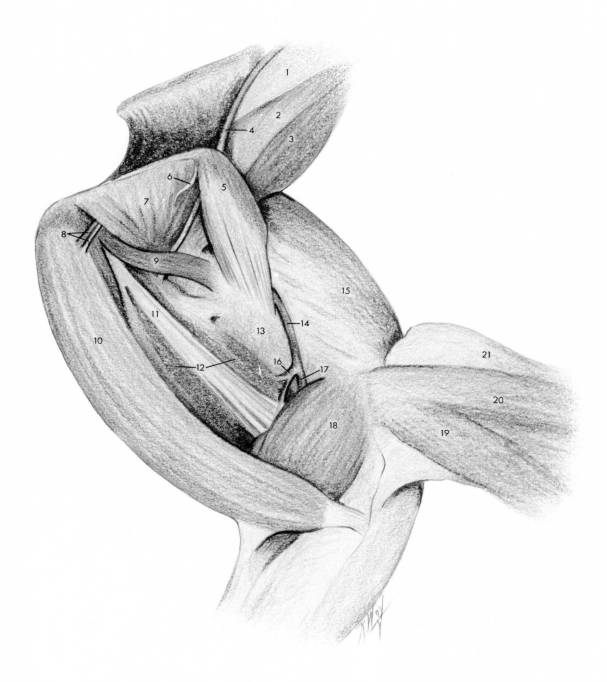

(Plate 82) 183

PLATE 83

Deep dissection of the sublumbar and the medial femoral muscles. The abductor muscle has been removed and the pectineus muscle reflected downward.

1. Psoas minor muscle
2. Psoas major muscle
3. Cranial portion of the iliacus muscle. The caudal portion is labeled 3a.
4. Branch of the obturator nerve which innervated the gracilis and abductor muscles, now reflected
5. Obturator externus muscle, which originates on the ventral surface of the pubis and ischium. It inserts in the trochanteric fossa of the femur.
6. Branches of the caudal gluteal nerve and artery to the semitendinosus muscle
7. Semitendinosus muscle
8. Quadratus femoris muscle
9. Sciatic nerve
10. Distal end of the pectineus muscle, which has been reflected downward
11. Medial head of the gastrocnemius muscle, which arises from the medial supracondyloid crest of the femur
12. Reflected gracilis, sartorius and semimembranosus muscles

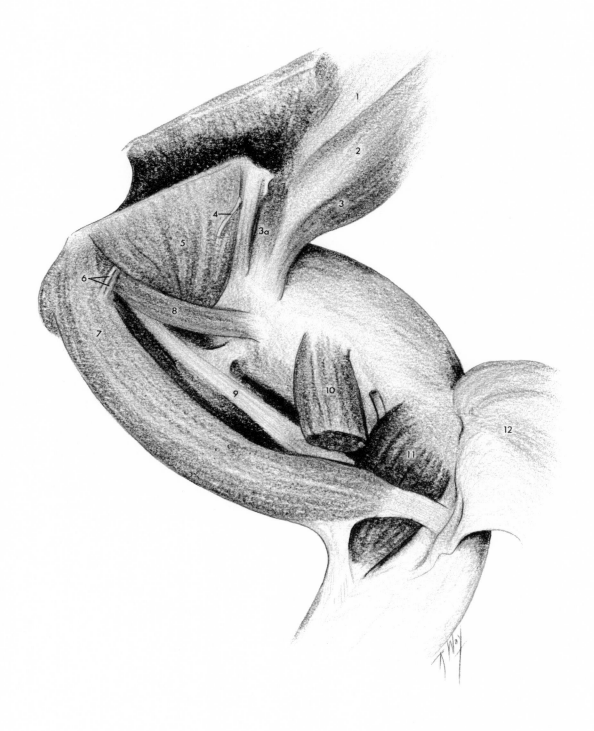

(Plate 83)   185

PLATE 84

A ventral view of the pelvis to illustrate the muscles and the ligaments associated with the hip joint. The capsule of the joint has been cut and the head of the femur removed to expose the acetabulum and the ligaments of the joint.

1. Prepubic tendon
2. Accessory ligament, present only in the equidae, which extends from the prepubic tendon through the acetabular notch to attach to the head of the femur. This ligament provides an especially firm anchorage for the head of the femur within the acetabulum.
3. Transverse ligament, which converts the ace-tabular notch into a foramen through which the accessory ligament extends
4. Reflected joint capsule
5. Acetabulum
6. The cotyloid ligament, which is attached to the bony margin of the acetabulum and serves to make it deeper
7. Tendon of insertion of the iliopsoas muscle
8. Quadriceps femoris muscle
9. Pectineus muscle, which has been detached from its origin and reflected downward
10. Deep face of the obturator externus muscle, which has been detached from its origin and reflected downward
11. Gamellus muscle, which arises from the lateral border of the ischium and inserts on the trochanteric fossa and ridge of the femur
12. Quadratus femoris, which has been cut from its insertion and reflected backward

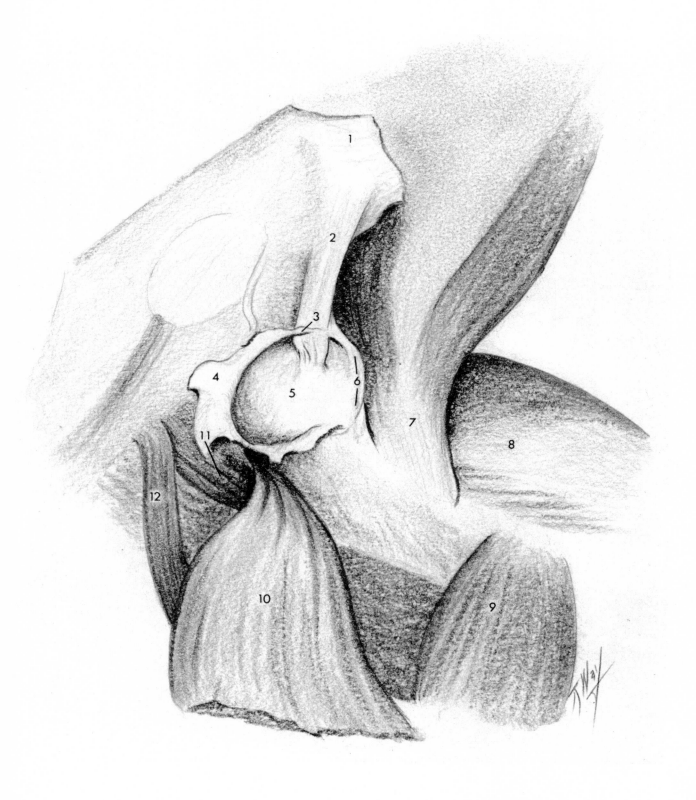

(Plate 84) 187

PLATE 85

This plate differs from the preceding one in that the iliopsoas muscle has been detached from its origin and reflected downward to illustrate to better advantage the heads of the quadriceps femoris.

1. Quadriceps femoris muscle
2. Rectus femoris head of the quadriceps, arising by means of two strong tendons from the shaft of the ilium
3. Vastus medialis head of the quadriceps, which arises from the medial surface of the femur
4. Deep face of the tendon of insertion of the iliopsoas

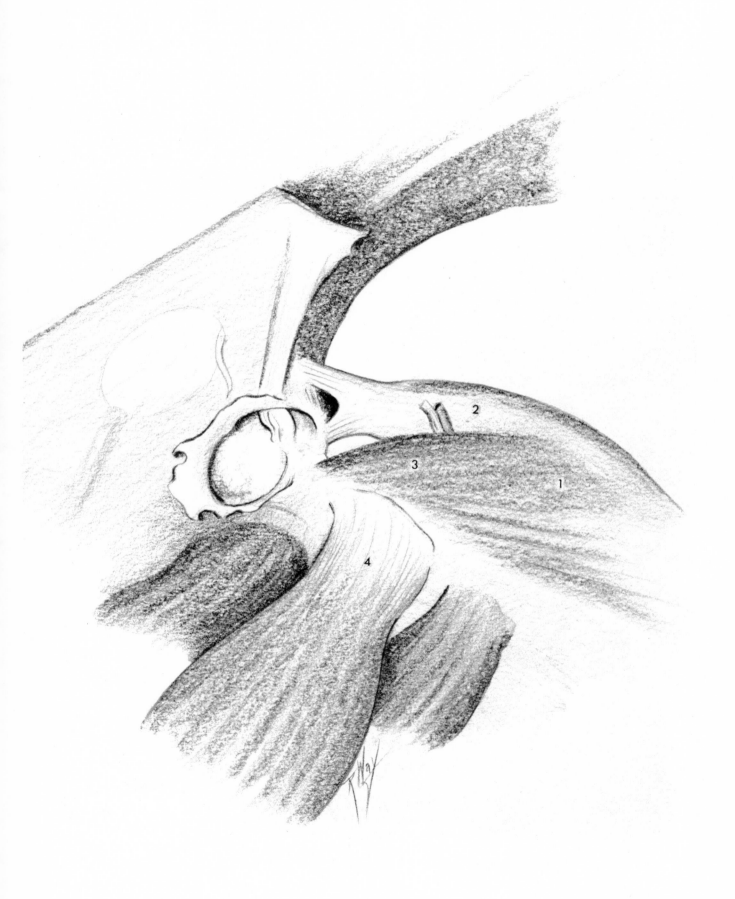

(Plate 85)   189

PLATE 86

A medial view of the muscles, the vessels and the nerves of the caudal tibial or leg region of the pelvic limb

1. Terminal portion of the sciatic nerve
2. Fibular, or peroneal, branch of the sciatic nerve
3. Muscular branch of the sciatic which divides into numerous branches which innervate the caudal tibial muscles
4. Proximal end of the tibial nerve
5. Medial surface of the distal end of the biceps femoris muscle
6. Medial head of the gastrocnemius muscle. Note that its tendon of insertion spirals lateral to the tendon of the superficial digital flexor tendon (10). Here it joins that of the lateral head and the common tendon continues distad to insert on the tuber calcis (6a).
7. The popliteus muscle attaching to the caudal surface of the tibia
8. Long digital flexor muscle, which is the medial head of the deep digital flexor
9. Flexor hallicis longus muscle, which is the deep head of the deep digital flexor
10. Superficial digital flexor
11. Recurrent tibial vein
12. Distal end of the tibial nerve. Note that it divides distally to form the medial and the lateral plantar nerves. A flap of deep fascia (12a) lies between the tibial nerve and the flexor hallicis longus muscle.
13. Distal end of the caudal tibial artery
14. Lateral tarsal artery, which passes downward on the lateral surface of the hock
15. Medial tarsal artery
16. Recurrent tibial branch of the medial tarsal artery

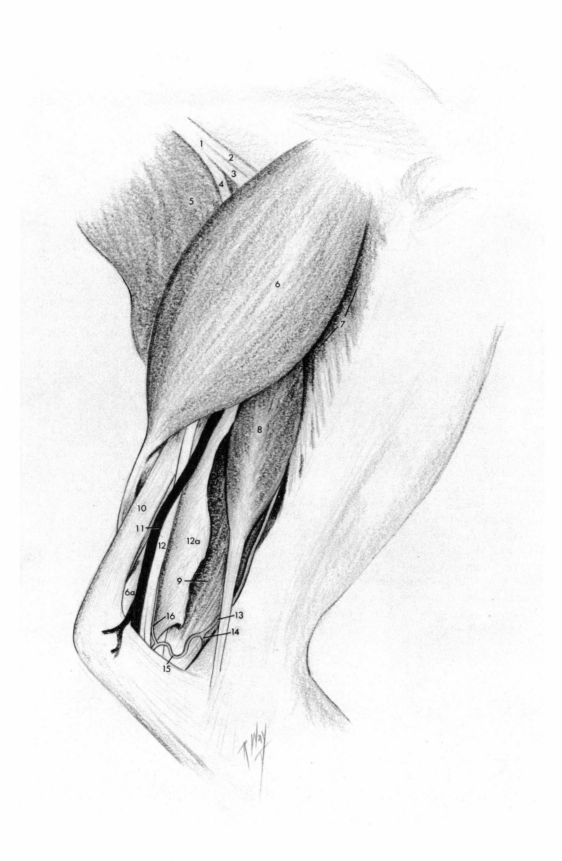

(Plate 86)   191

PLATE 87

This view is similar to the preceding plate, but the origin of the medial head of the gastrocnemius muscle has been cut and the muscle reflected caudad to permit a deeper view.

1. Reflected medial head of the gastrocnemius
2. Sciatic nerve
3. Tibial nerve
4. Muscular branch of the sciatic which ramifies to innervate all of the caudal tibial muscles
5. Fibular, or peroneal, nerve which passes lateral to the lateral head of the gastrocnemius (10)
6. Distal end of the femoral artery
7. Popliteal artery, which passes between the two heads of the gastrocnemius muscle and then dips beneath the popliteus muscle and divides into cranial and the caudal tibial arteries
8. Distal caudal femoral artery
9. Superficial digital flexor muscle, which originates from the supracondyloid fossa of the femur. Its tendon of insertion passes distad to the point of the hock where it widens to cover the tuber calcis (9a). Some fibers attach to the tuber calcis. Others continue distad as a strong rounded tendon (9b) to the digit. The superficial digital flexor of the horse is largely tendinous and thus its action is predominantly mechanical. It acts mechanically to extend the hock when the stifle is extended (the opposite of the peroneus tertius) and to provide mechanical support for the fetlock.
10. Lateral head of the gastrocnemius, which originates from the lateral supracondyloid crest of the femur
11. Popliteus muscle
12. Long digital flexor muscle
13. Flexor hallucis longus muscle
14. Tibialis caudalis muscle. (12), (13), and (14) are the three muscular heads of the deep digital flexor muscle. Their tendons converge below the hock to form a single tendon which extends to the digit.
15. Caudal tibial artery
16. Lateral tarsal artery
17. Medial tarsal artery
18. Recurrent tibial branch of the medial tarsal artery. Note that this is directly continuous in this specimen (as is frequently true) with the descending branch of (8).

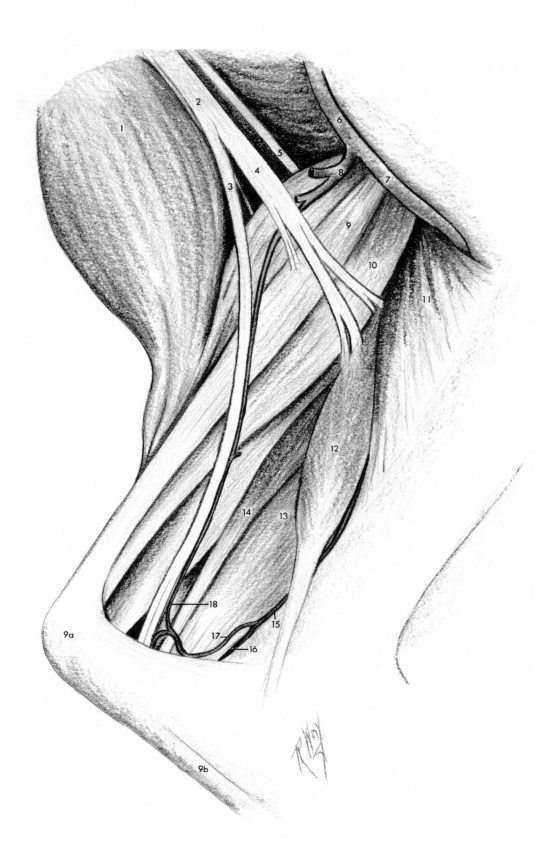

(Plate 87)   193

PLATE 88

The dorsolateral muscles of the leg, cranial view.

1. Long digital extensor muscle, which originates above from the extensor fossa of the femur. Its long tendon of insertion (1a) extends downward to the foot and is further illustrated in Plate 91.
2. Lateral digital extensor muscle, which arises from the lateral ligament of the stifle joint, the fibula and the lateral border of the tibia. Its long tendon (2a) extends downward below the hock and joins the tendon of the long extensor.
3. Peroneus tertius—a muscle in most species of animals, but in the equidae reduced to a powerful ligament extending from the extensor fossa of the femur downward to split into two ligaments. The lateral one of these (3a) inserts on the fibular and the 4th tarsal bones. The medial one (3b) spirals beneath the tendon of insertion of the tibialis cranialis muscle (4a) to attach to the proximal end of the large metacarpal bone. Whenever the stifle joint is flexed, the peroneus tertius mechanically flexes the hock. For this reason the horse cannot flex his stifle without simultaneously flexing his hock.
4. Tibialis cranialis muscle, which originates from the lateral condyle and border of the tibia. Its tendon of insertion (4a) passes between the medial and the lateral ligaments of attachment of the peroneus tertius and then divides into medial and lateral tendons. The medial one (sometimes termed the cunean tendon) attaches to the 1st tarsal bone and the lateral one attaches to the large metatarsal bone.
5. Cranial surface of the tibia
6. Proximal annular ligament
7. Middle annular ligament
8. Distal annular ligament
9. Proximal end of the large or third metatarsal bone

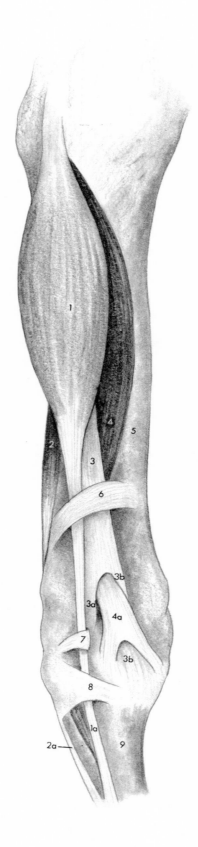

(Plate 88)   195

PLATE 89

This plate differs only slightly from the preceding. The peroneus tertius is shown in its entirety; this has been accomplished by severing the tendon of insertion of the long extensor muscle and reflecting the muscular head laterad.

1. Long extensor and (1a) its tendon of insertion at point of severance
2. Peroneus tertius, nothing more than a wide flat ligament adherent to the cranial face of (3).
3. Tibialis cranialis muscle
4. Lateral digital extensor muscle
5. Extensor digitalis brevis muscle, a vestigial muscle of little importance in the horse
6. Point of union of the tendons of insertion of the long and the lateral digital extensor muscles

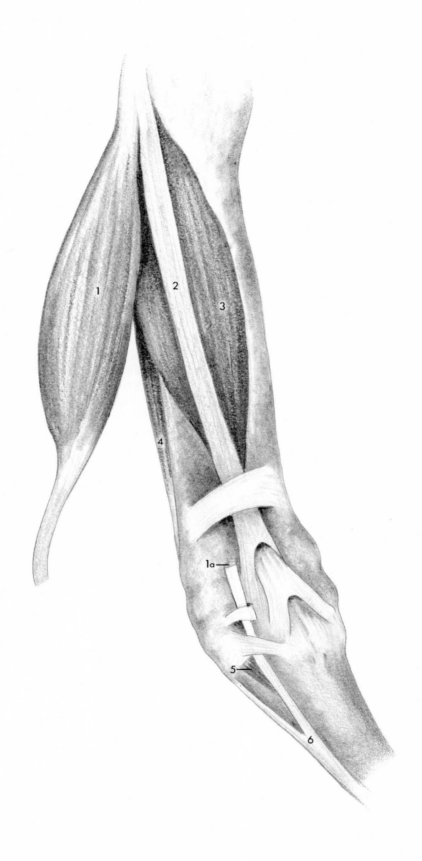

(Plate 89)   197

PLATE 90

In this plate all of the dorsolateral muscles of the leg have been severed in order to expose the cranial tibial artery.

1. Reflected long digital extensor and (1a) its tendon of insertion
2. Lateral digital extensor
3. Proximal end and distal end (3a) of the peroneus tertius
4. The proximal muscular head of the tibialis cranialis and its tendon of insertion (4a)
5. Fibula
6. Cranial tibial artery, which is the largest terminal of the popliteal artery. It runs forward through the interosseous space between the tibia and the fibula, then descends obliquely over the cranial surface of the tibia to reach the hock. Here it gives off the perforating tarsal artery (6a) and is continued as the great metatarsal artery (6b). These terminals lie beneath the extensor digitalis brevis muscle which has been removed to illustrate them.

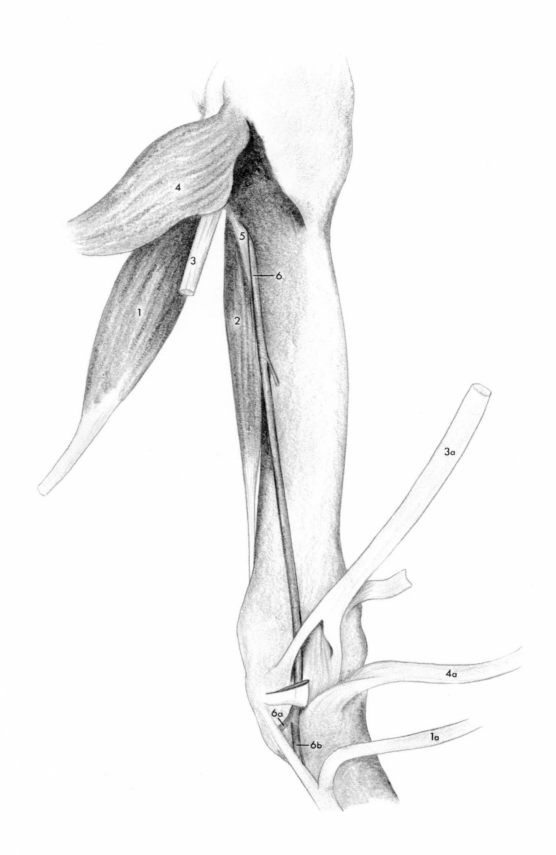

(Plate 90)   199

PLATE 91

A cranial view of the ligaments and the tendons of the right tarsus, metatarsus and digit of the pelvic limb

1. Proximal annular ligament
2. Middle annular ligament
3. Distal annular ligament
4. Lateral malleolus of the tibia
5. Medial malleolus of the tibia
6. Medial ridge of the trochlea of the tibial tarsal bone
7. Tendon of insertion of the tibialis cranialis muscle. Its medial branch (cunean tendon) can be seen extending medially to attach to the first tarsal bone.
8. Tendon of the long digital extensor muscle
9. Tendon of the lateral digital extensor muscle
10. Lateral and medial (10a) branches of the interosseous medius or suspensory ligament of the fetlock
11. Third metatarsal bone
12. First phalanx (long pastern)
13. Second phalanx (short pastern)
14. Third phalanx (coffin bone)

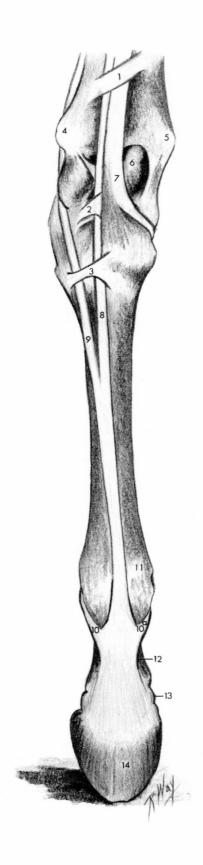

(Plate 91)   201

PLATE 92

A medial view of the bones of the pelvic limb illustrating the relative position of the principal arteries. The solid arteries are medial to the bones, whereas those that are in dotted lines are situated in a lateral position.

1. Terminal end of the aorta
2. Internal iliac or hypogastric artery
3. Iliolumbar artery
4. Umbilical artery
5. Lateral sacral artery
6. Cranial gluteal artery
7. Internal pudendal artery
8. Iliaco-femoral artery
9. Obturator artery. (8) and (9) are terminals of the internal iliac artery.
10. External iliac artery
11. Pudendo-epigastric or prepubic artery
12. Femoral artery
13. Deep femoral artery
14. Saphenous artery
15. The distal caudal femoral artery
16. Popliteal artery
17. Caudal tibial artery
18. Cranial tibial artery
19. Medial tarsal artery
20. Recurrent tibial artery
21. Lateral tarsal artery
22. Recurrent tarsal artery
23. The medial and the lateral plantar arteries
24. Proximal plantar arch
25. Perforating tarsal artery
26. Great metatarsal artery
27. Medial and lateral superficial plantar metatarsal arteries
28. Medial and lateral deep plantar metatarsals
29. Division of the great metatarsal artery into medial and lateral proper digital arteries. Note the union of the superficial and the deep plantar metatarsal arteries with the digital arteries. This union forms the distal plantar arch. However, the arrangement of vessels here is quite variable.
30. Medial and lateral proper digital arteries
31. Artery of the 1st phalanx
32. Artery of the 2nd phalanx
33. Terminal arch formed by anastomosis of the medial and the lateral proper digital arteries within the semilunar canal of the os pedis
    A. Sacrum
    B. Os coxae or hip bone
    C. Femur
    D. Patella
    E. Tibia
    F. Tarsus
    G. Metatarsus
    H. First phalanx or long pastern
    I. Second phalanx or short pastern
    J. Third phalanx or os pedis

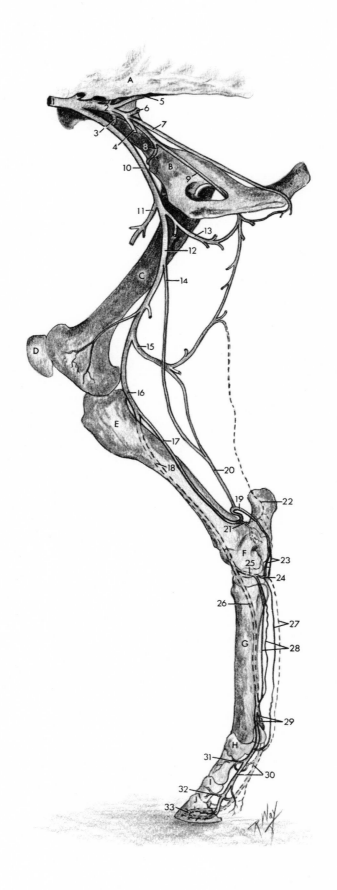

(Plate 92)   203

PLATE 93

The veins of the pelvic limb — medial view

1. Middle dorsal metatarsal vein
2. Medial dorsal metatarsal vein
3. Medial and lateral superficial plantar metatarsal veins
4. Deep plantar metatarsal vein
5. Cranial tibial vein
6. Caudal tibial vein
7. Recurrent tibial vein and (7a) the anastomosis between the recurrent tibial vein and the caudal ramus of the medial saphenous vein
8. Recurrent tarsal vein
9. Cranial ramus of the medial saphenous vein
10. Caudal ramus of the medial saphenous vein
11. Medial saphenous vein
12. Popliteal vein
13. Caudal femoral vein
14. Femoral vein

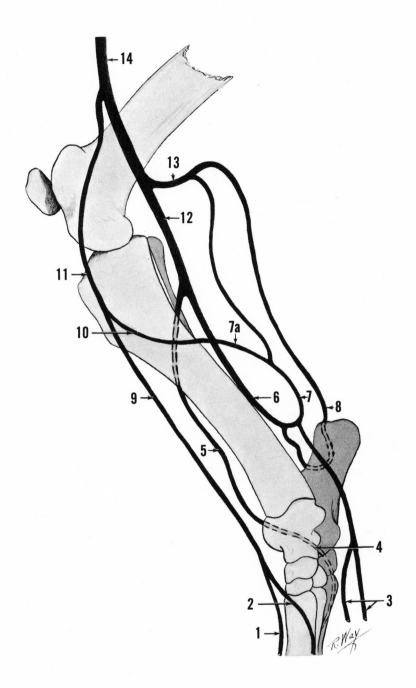

(Plate 93) 205

INDEX

Acetabulum, femoral, 38
  of hip joint, 140, 142, 144, 186
Alveoli, 6
Antebrachium *See* Shoulder.
Anus, 60, 165, 168
Aorta, abdominal, 50
  terminal bifurcation, 50
  terminus, 202
  thoracic, 44, 46
Aponeurosis, brachiocephalicus, 92
  conjoined, of brachiocephalicus and superficial pec-
    toral muscles, 112
  of external oblique abdominus, 30, 38
  of internal oblique abdominus, 40
  of rectus abdominus, 30
  of transversus abdominus muscle, 50
Arch, costal, 40, 48
  distal volar, 120, 122
  ischial, 56, 142
  proximal plantar, 202
  proximal volar, 120, 122
  terminal, 120, 202
Arm, 28
Artery(ies), angular, 10
  axillary, 44, 100, 106, 109
  brachial, 100, 109
  brachiocephalic, 44
  carouid, 46
  caudal circumflex humeral, 100, 102, 104
  caudal deep epigastric, 40, 50
  caudal femoral, 182
  caudal gluteal, 166, 168, 182, 184
  caudal tibial, 190, 192, 202
  caudal superficial epigastric, 58
  circumflex iliac, 38, 40
  circumflex scapular, 100, 102, 104
  collateral ulnar, 100, 112, 114
  common brachio-cephalic, 46
  common carotid, 44
  common digital (medial superficial volar metacarpal),
    100, 116, 118, 120, 122, 130
  common interosseous, 100, 104
  common trunk, 176
  costocervical, 44, 46
  cranial circumflex humeral, 104
  cranial dorsal, of penis, 58
  cranial gluteal, 170, 172, 202
  cranial tibial, 198, 202
  deep brachial, 100, 104, 109
  deep circumflex, 172
    iliac, 50

Artery(ies) — (*Cont.*)
  deep cervical, 46
  deep femoral, 176, 202
  deep volar metacarpal, 114
  of digital cushion, 120
  distal caudal femoral, 202
  distal collateral radial, 100, 104
  dorsal interosseous, 104
  dorsal metacarpal, 120
  external iliac, 38, 172, 176, 180, 182, 202
  external maxillary, 12
  external pudendal, 40, 58
  external thoracic, 46
  facial, 10
  femoral, 176, 180, 182, 192, 202
  of 1st phalanx, 120, 202
  gluteal, 165
  great metatarsal, 202
  hypogastric, 172, 202
  iliacofemoral, 170, 172, 202
  iliolumbar, 170, 202
  inferior labial, 10
  intercostal, 44
  internal iliac, 172, 202
  internal pudendal, 168, 170, 172, 202
  internal thoracic, 44, 46
  lateral coccygeal, 168
  lateral deep plantar metacarpal, 202
  lateral deep volar metacarpal, 100, 118, 120, 122
  lateral distal, 130
  lateral nasal, 10
  lateral plantar, 202
  lateral proper digital, 120, 202
  lateral sacral, 168, 172, 202
  lateral superficial plantar metatarsal, 202
  lateral tarsal, 190, 192, 202
  left axillary, 46
  left common carotid, 46
  left coronary, circumflex branch, 46
    descending branch, 46
  left subclavian, 46
  masseteric, 10
  medial deep plantar metacarpal, 202
  medial deep volar metacarpal, 100, 114, 118, 120, 122
  medial dorsal metacarpal, 116
  medial plantar, 202
  medial proper digital, 116, 120, 202
  medial superficial plantar metatarsal, 202
  medial superficial volar metacarpal (common digital),
    100
  medial tarsal, 190, 202
  median, 100, 114, 116, 118, 120
  middle deep volar metacarpal, 122
  midline uterine, 60
  obturator, 38, 166, 170, 172, 202
  omocervical, 44, 46

Artery(ies) — (Cont.)
  perforating tarsal, 202
  phrenic, 46
  popliteal, 180, 182, 198, 202
  prepubic, 40, 176, 202
  proper digital, 122
  pudendal, 166
  pudendo-epigastric, 202
  pulmonary, 46
  recurrent tarsal, 202
  recurrent tibial, 202
  of rete carpi volare, 100, 116, 118
  saphenous, 202
  of 2nd phalanx, 120, 202
  subscapular, 100, 102, 108
  superficial volar metacarpal, 116, 118, 120
  superior labial, 10
  suprascapular, 100, 109
  tarsal, 198
  of 3rd phalanx, 120
  thoracodorsal, 100, 109, 112
  transverse facial, 10
  ulnar, 110, 114, 116, 120
  umbilical, 60, 172, 202
  utero-ovarian, 60
  vertebral, 44, 46
Articulation, sacrosciatic, 140
Atlas, 6, 14
Ausus, 174
Axis, 6

Bladder, urinary, 50, 54, 60
Bone(s), accessory carpal, 74, 76, 116, 120
  cannon See Bone, 3rd metatarsal.
  carpus, 66
  central tarsal, 150
  clavicle, 82
  coffin See Bone, 3rd phalanx.
  distal sesamoid, 66, 76, 134
  dorsal turbinate, 14
  ethmoturbinates, 14
  femur, 64, 146, 154, 156, 162, 180, 182, 186, 188, 194,
    202
  fibula, 64, 148, 154, 156, 158, 198
    tarsal, 150, 152
  5th sacral vertebra, 142
  1st carpal, 74, 76
  1st phalanx (long pastern), 64, 66, 76, 82, 96, 124, 128,
    134, 202
  1st sacral vertebra, 140
  4th carpal, 74, 76
  4th or lateral metatarsal (splint), 64
  4th metacarpal, 76, 82
  frontal, 6
    supraorbital process, 6
  hip, 202
  humerus, 24, 48, 66, 68, 70, 82, 86, 94, 96, 98, 104, 110
    lateral condyle, 70
    medial condyle, 70
  hyoid, 14
  ilium, 64, 140, 170, 176, 188
  incisive See Premaxilla.
  intermediate carpal, 74, 76
  ischium, 64, 140, 166, 180, 182, 184
  lacrimal, 6
  large metacarpal See Bone, 3rd metacarpal.

Bone(s) — (Cont.)
  lateral metacarpal See Bone, 4th metatarsal.
  lateral proximal sesamoid, 64, 76
  lateral small metacarpal, 122
  lateral splint, 76
  long pastern See Bone, 1st phalanx.
  mandible, 6, 14
    coronoid process, 6
  mandibular, 12
  maxilla, 6
  medial metacarpal See Bone, 2nd metacarpal.
  medial metatarsal See Bone, 2nd metatarsal.
  medial sesamoid, 76
  medial splint, 76
  metacarpal, 66
  metatarsal, 152, 200, 202
  nasal, 6
  navicular, 66, 76, 134
  occipital, 6
  parietal, 6
  patella, 64, 154, 158, 202
  phalanx, 200, 202
  premaxilla, 6, 14
  proximal sesamoid, 66
  pubic, 50, 64, 140, 172, 176, 180, 184
  radial carpal, 74, 76
  radius, 48, 64, 66, 72, 76, 86, 92, 94, 96, 98, 104, 112
  rib, 176
  sacrum, 140, 202
  scapula, 48, 64, 66, 68, 82, 94, 98, 102, 104, 110
  2nd carpal, 74, 76
  2nd metacarpal, 76, 82, 94
  2nd metatarsal, 64
  2nd phalanx, 64, 66, 76, 96, 130, 134, 202
  sesamoid, 122, 128, 130
  tarsal, 64, 150, 152, 194, 202
  temporal, 6
    petrous portion, 6
    squamous portion, 6
  thigh, 64
  3rd carpal, 74, 76
  3rd metacarpal, 66, 116, 134
  3rd metatarsal, 64, 150
  3rd phalanx, 64, 66, 76, 124, 128, 200
  tibia, 64, 148, 162, 190, 194, 198, 202
  tibial tarsal, 150, 152
  ulna, 48, 64, 66, 72, 82, 86, 94, 96, 98, 104
  ulnar carpal, 74, 76
  ventral turbinate, 14
  zygomatic, 6
Border, coronary, of hoof, 134
Bronchus, left, 46
Bursa, 134
  navicular, 134
  beneath tendon of infraspinatus muscle, 104
  of tendon of lateral digital extensor, 126
  trochanteric, 170

Caecum, 48
Canal, carpal, 116
  sacral, 140, 142
  semilunar, of os pedis, 202
  vascular, of tarsus, 150
Cap, knee, 64
Capsule, of fetlock joint, 126, 134
  of hip joint, 186

Cartilage, accessory of 3rd phalanx, 126
  cariniform, 92
  costal, 36, 90
  cricoid, 14
  scapular, 68, 84
  thyroid, 14
Cavity, abdominal, 48
  of coffin joint, 134
  cranial, 8
  of fetlock joint, 134
  glenoid, 68, 70, 102
  nasal, 8
  oral, 14
  orbital, 8
  of pastern joint, 134
  pelvic, 50, 166, 176
  thoracic, 48
Cerebellum, 14
Cleft, vulvar, 60
Colon, descending, 48
  great, 48
  small, 48
Condyle, femoral, 156, 158
  lateral, 194
  lateral femoral, 154
  lateral tibial, 148, 154
  tibial, 156, 158
Cord, spermatic, 50
   left, 54
   right, 54
Corium, coronary, 134
  of frog, 134
  laminar, 116, 134
  of sole, 134
Cornua, uterine, 60
Corpus cavernosus urethrae, 56
Crest, condyloid, of humerus, 102, 104
  humeral, 82, 104, 112
  of ilium, 140, 142
  lateral condyloid, of humerus, 82
  supracondyloid, of femur, 184
  tibial, 162
  trochanteric, 146
Crura, penile, 56
Cushion, digital, 134
  distal, 128

Diaphragm, 44, 48
  pelvic, 168
Digit(s), 66
Duct, great lymphatic, 46
  great thoracic lymph, 44
  parotid salivary gland, 12
Ductus deferens, left, 54
  right, 54

Elbow, 86, 104, 108
Eminence, iliopectineal, 140
  median, of pubic bones, 50
Epicondyle, lateral, of humerus, 104
  of femur, 146
  medial, of femur, 146, 178
   of humerus, 94, 96, 112, 114
Epiglottis, 14
Ergot, 116, 134

Esophagus, 14, 44, 46
External auditory meatus, 6

Fascia, antebrachial, 114
  coccygeal, 162
  crural, 176, 178
  deep antebrachial, 94
  gluteal, 162
  lata, 162
Fetlock, 116
  suspensory ligament, 96, 98
Fold, genital, 50, 54
  vocal, 14
Foramen, infraorbital, 6
  lesser sciatic, 166
  obturator, 140, 144
Forearm, 109
Fossa, extensor, of femur, 146, 194
  infraspinatus, 68
  infraspinous, 88, 102
   of scapula, 86
  intercondyloid, 146
  olecranon, 70
  subscapular, 68, 94
  supracondyloid, of femur, 146, 192
  supraspinatus, 68
  supraspinous, of scapula, 86
  trochanteric, 146
   of femur, 184
Frog, of hoof, 128, 134

Girdle, pelvic, 64, 140
Gland, bulbo-urethral, 54
  internal iliac lymph, 50
  parotid salivary, 12
  thyroid, 46
Groove, musculospiral, 86
  of humerus, 102, 104

Head, 1–15
Heart, 44, 46, 48
Hemisphere, left cerebral, 14
Hock, 150, 190
Hoof, 134
Horn, uterine, 60

Ilium, 38
Impact, absorption, 20
Interosseous medius, 116, 124, 130, 200
Intestine, small, 48

Joint, coffin, 134
  fetlock, 134
  hip, 186
  pastern, 130, 134
  shoulder, 70
  stifle, 154, 156, 158, 180, 194

Kidney, 60
"Knee," 64, 66

Lacertus fibrosus, 136
Larynx, 14
  lateral ventricle, 14
Leg, 64
Ligament(s), accessory, 176, 186
   of hip joint, 38

Ligament(s)—(Cont.)
  bladder, middle, 50
  broad, 60
  caudal cruciate, 146, 148
  caudal, of medial meniscus, 148
  central volar of pastern joint, 128
  condyloid, 186
  cranial cruciate, 146, 148
  cranial, of lateral meniscus, 148, 156
    of medial meniscus, 148
  distal annular, 194, 200
  distal digital annular, 128
  dorsal sacroiliac, 162, 164, 168
  of ergot, 116
  femoral, 146
    of lateral meniscus, 156
  femoro-tibial, 146
  inferior check, 96, 98
  intersesamoidean, 130, 134
  lateral collateral, of elbow, 104
  lateral cruciate, 156
  lateral, of elbow, 104
  lateral femoro-patellar, 154
  lateral femoro-tibial, 148, 154, 156, 158
  lateral patellar, 154, 158, 162
  lateral sacroiliac, 144, 162, 164, 168, 170
  medial collateral, 112
    of elbow, 114
  medial cruciate, 156
  medial femoro-tibial, 146, 148, 156, 158
  medial patellar, 154, 158
  middle annular, 194, 200
  middle distal sesamoidean, 128, 130
  middle patellar, 154, 158
  middle sesamoidean, 134
  patellar, 148
  peroneus tertius, 194, 196, 198
  proximal annular, 194, 200
  proximal digital annular, 126, 128, 130
  round, 60
  sacroiliac, 166
  sacrosciatic, 144, 166, 168, 170, 178
  superficial sesamoidean, 134
  superficial distal sesamoidean, 130
  superior check, 72, 96
  superior sesamoidean, 130
  supraspinatus, 36, 84
  supraspinous, 82, 90
  suspensory, of anus, 174
    of distal sesamoid, 134
    of elbow, 76
    of fetlock, 116, 120, 122, 124, 130, 136, 152, 200
      abaxial branch, 128
    of navicular bone, 128
  transverse, 186
  volar annular, of fetlock, 126, 128
  volar, of carpus, 96
    of pastern joint, 130
  volar transverse, of carpus, 116
Ligamentum nuchae, 14, 32, 34, 36
Limb, front, 66
  pelvic, 202, 204
Line, gluteal, 142
  iliopectineal, 140
Lung, basal border, 48
  cardiac notch, 48

Lung—(Cont.)
  left, 36
  parietal surface, 48

Malleolus, lateral, of tibia, 200
  medial, of tibia, 200
Mandible, 6
  coronoid process, 6
Meatus, dorsal nasal, 14
  inferior nasal, 14
  middle nasal, 14
Medulla oblongata, 14
Meniscus, lateral, 146, 154, 156, 158
  medial, 156, 158
Mesorchium, 50
Mesorectum, 50
Muscle(s), abdominal, oblique, 50
  abductor, 182
  accessory gluteal, 164
  adductor, 146, 166, 178, 180
    femoris, 144
  anconeus, 70, 72, 86, 102, 104
  biceps brachii, 68, 72, 84, 86, 88, 92, 94, 96, 106, 108, 112, 114
  biceps femoris, 24, 144, 146, 148, 152, 166, 180, 182, 190
  biceps major, 162
  brachialis, 70, 72, 86, 88, 92, 96, 98, 102, 104, 112
  brachiocephalicus, 4, 12, 24, 26, 28, 70, 82, 84, 88, 92, 102, 104
  buccinator, 4
  capsularis, 38, 68, 70, 144, 146
  caudal deep pectoral, 24, 28, 70, 82, 88, 90, 94, 104, 106
  caudal superficial pectoral, 28, 92
  caudal tibial, 148, 192
  coccygeus, 162, 165, 168, 174
  common digital extensor, 70, 72, 82, 104, 124
  common digital flexor, 76
  constrictor vestibuli, 60
  constrictor vulvae, 60
  coracobrachialis, 68, 70, 94, 96, 98, 108
  cranial deep pectoral, 26, 28, 82, 84, 86, 90, 94, 110
  cranial superficial pectoral, 28, 82, 88, 92
  cranial tibial, 148
  crescentic, 165
  cutaneous colli, 24, 32, 92
  cutaneous omobrachialis, 88
  deep digital flexor, 70, 72, 76, 82, 96, 98, 104, 118, 152
  deep pectoral, 90
  deltoideus, 24, 68, 70, 82, 84, 102
  depressor labii inferioris, 4
  digital flexor, 192
  dilatator naris lateralis, 4
  extensor carpi obliquus, 72, 76, 82, 86, 104, 124
  extensor carpi radialis, 70, 76, 82, 92, 94, 102, 104, 112, 116, 124, 136
  extensor carpi ulnaris, 118
  extensor digitalis brevis, 196, 198
  external anal sphincter, 174
  external cremaster, 40, 56
  external intercostal, 26
  external oblique abdominus, 24, 28, 38
  external obturator, 144, 146, 170, 182, 184, 186
  flexor carpi lateralis, 76
  flexor carpi radialis, 70, 76, 92, 94, 112, 114
  flexor carpi ulnaris, 70, 72, 94, 112, 114, 116

Muscle(s)—(*Cont.*)

flexor hallicus, 148
  longus, 190, 192
fronto-scutularis, 4
fusiform, 112
fusiform capsularis, 102
fusiform ventral sacroccygeus, 174
gamellus, 144, 146, 170, 186
gastrocnemius, 146, 152, 156, 178, 180, 182, 184, 190, 192
genioglosseus, 14
geniohyoideus, 14
gluteus medius, 24, 144, 146, 162, 164, 170
gluteus profundus, 144, 146, 164
gluteus superficialis, 24, 144, 146, 162
gracilis, 56, 58, 144, 148, 176, 178, 180, 184
human deltoideus, 4
human sterno-cleidomastoideus, 4
hyoepiglotticus, 14
iliacus, 38, 40, 172, 176, 180, 182, 184
iliocostalis, 30, 32, 34
iliopsoas, 146, 176, 186
infraspinatus, 26, 68, 70, 84, 86, 102, 104, 106
internal oblique abdominus, 32, 40
internal obturator, 146, 166
interosseous, 76
interosseous medius, 96, 136, 152
intertransversales caudae, 162, 165, 168
intertransversarii, 34
ischiocavernosus, 56, 174
lateral digital extensor, 72, 76, 82, 88, 104, 148, 194, 198
lateral sacrococcygeus, 168
lateral volar metacarpal, 118
latissimus dorsi, 24, 82, 90, 94, 102, 106, 108
levatores costarum, 36
levator labii superioris, 4
levator labii superioris proprius, 4
levator nasiolabialis, 4
long digital extensor, 146, 154, 190, 194, 198
long digital flexor, 148
longissimus atlantis, 32
longissimus capitis, 32
longissimus cervicis, 30, 32
longissimus dorsi, 30, 32, 34
longitudinal lingual, 14
masseter, 4
medial interosseous, 122
mentalis, 4
multifidis cervicis, 34
multifidis dorsi, 36, 50, 168
multifidis lumborum, 36
mylohyoideus, 12, 14
nasolabialis, 4
obliquus abdominus internus *See* Muscle, internal oblique abdominus.
obliquus capitis cranialis, 34
obturator externus *See* Muscle, external obturator.
obturator internus *See* Muscle, internal obturator.
omohyoideus, 12, 110
orbicularis oris, 4
parotido-auricularis, 4
pectineus, 144, 146, 176, 178, 180, 182, 184, 186
periformis, 146
peroneus tertius, 146, 152, 154
plantaris, 146
popliteus, 146, 148, 190, 192

Muscle(s)—(*Cont.*)

prepubic, 176
pronator teres, 112, 114
psoas major, 50, 172, 176, 178, 180, 182, 184
psoas minor, 38, 50, 172, 176, 178, 180, 182, 184
  tendon, 38
quadratus femoris, 144, 146, 166, 170, 182, 184, 186
quadriceps femoris, 176, 178, 180, 182, 186, 188
rectococcygeus, 60, 174
rectus abdominus, 30, 32, 34, 50
rectus capitis dorsalis, 14
rectus capitis ventralis, 14
rectus capitis ventralis major, 32, 34
rectus femoris, 38, 144, 170, 172, 188
rectus thoracis, 30, 32, 34
retractor ani, 168
retractor penis, 56, 174
rhomboideus, 68, 84, 88
rhomboideus cervicalis, 24, 26, 28, 94
rhomboideus thoracalis, 26, 28
sacrococcygeus dorsalis, 162, 168
sacrococcygeus lateralis, 162
sacrococcygeus ventralis, 162
sartorius, 176, 178, 180, 182, 184
scalenus, 32, 106
semimembranosus, 56, 58, 144, 146, 162, 166, 170, 178, 180, 182, 184
semispinalis capitis, 32
semispinalis dorsi, 34
semitendinosus, 24, 144, 148, 152, 162, 166, 170, 176, 178, 180, 182, 184
serratus dorsalis caudalis, 26
serratus dorsalis cranialis, 26
serratus ventralis, 68, 82, 84, 88, 106
serratus ventralis cervicis, 24, 26, 28
serratus ventralis thoracis, 24, 26, 28, 136
sphincter ani, 168
spinalis, 34
spinalis et semispinalis, 32
splenius, 24, 28, 30, 44
sternocephalicus, 4, 12, 30, 32
sternohyoideus, 12, 14
sterno-thyro-hyoideus, 34
subscapularis, 70, 94, 106, 108, 112
superficial digital flexor, 70, 72, 76, 96, 116, 118, 136, 146, 152, 190, 192
superficial gluteal, 164
superficial, of head, 4
superficial pectoral, 104
suprascapularis, 108
supraspinatus, 26, 68, 70, 84, 86, 94, 102, 104, 106, 110
tensor fasciae antebrachii, 72, 94, 102, 109, 112
tensor fasciae latae, 24, 144, 162, 164, 165, 170
teres major, 68, 94, 102, 108, 112
teres minor, 68, 70, 86, 88, 104
tibialis caudalis, 192
tibialis cranialis, 152, 194, 196, 198
transversus abdominus, 34, 36
  aponeurosis, 34
  tendon, 34
transversus costarum *See* Muscle, rectus thoracis.
trapezius, 44, 82
trapezius cervicalis, 24, 68
trapezius thoracalis, 24
triceps brachii, 24, 26, 68, 70, 72, 82, 84, 94, 98, 102, 104, 110, 112

Muscle(s)—(*Cont.*)
　ulnaris lateralis, 70, 76, 82, 86, 104, 118
　vastus intermedius, 146
　vastus lateralis, 146, 164, 170
　vastus medialis, 146, 172, 188
　ventral sacrococcygeus, 165, 168
　ventral sacrococcygeus medialis, 174
　zygomasticus, 4

Neck, 24
Nerve(s), axillary, 112
　axillary, 80, 92, 102, 104, 106, 108
　caudal auricular, 10
　caudal cutaneous femoral, 170, 172
　caudal gluteal, 165, 168, 170, 172, 184
　caudal hemorrhoidal, 168, 172, 174
　cranial, 168
　cranial cutaneous antebrachial, 92, 102
　cranial gluteal, 164, 165, 170, 172
　cutaneous, 80
　　of neck, 10
　digital, 116
　dorsal esophageal, 44
　8th cervical, 80, 106
　external spermatic, 40, 58
　external thoracic, 106, 109
　facial, 10
　　auriculo-palpebral branch, 10
　femoral, 38, 172
　fibular, 180, 192
　1st thoracic, 106
　intercostal, 44
　intercostobracheal, 80
　lateral cutaneous, 38
　　of thigh, 40
　lateral volar metacarpal, 80, 116
　left dorsal, of penis, 58
　lumbar, 172
　medial cutaneous antebrachial, 92
　medial tarsal, 192
　medial volar metacarpal, 80, 116, 118
　median, 106, 108, 112, 114, 116
　metacarpal, 116
　musculocutaneous, 80, 92, 106, 108
　obturator, 38, 172, 180, 182, 184
　pelvic, 172
　peroneal, 170, 192
　phrenic, 44, 106
　pudendal, 168, 170, 172
　pulmonary, 46
　radial, 80, 102, 104, 106, 108, 112
　recurrent laryngeal, 44, 46
　sacral, 172
　saphenous, 176
　sciatic, 165, 166, 170, 172, 180, 182, 184, 190, 192
　2nd cervical, 10
　2nd intercostal, 80
　2nd sacral, 168
　7th cervical, 80, 106
　6th cervical, 80, 106
　spinal accessory, 44
　subscapular, 104, 106, 108
　suprascapular, 102, 106, 108
　suprascapularis, 109
　3rd cervical, 10

Nerve(s)—(*Cont.*)
　thoracic, 80, 106
　thoracodorsal, 108
　thoracodorsalis, 106
　tibial, 170, 180, 190, 192
　transverse facial, 10
　ulnar, 80, 106, 108, 112, 116, 118
　vagus, 44
　　combined with portion sympathetic trunk, 46
　　dorsal esophageal branch, 46
　　ventral esophageal branch, 46
　ventral esophageal, 44
　ventral thoracic, 80
　volar metacarpal, 116
Nervus transversarius, 46
Node, anal lymph, 168
　axillary lymph, 110
　cubital lymph, 110, 114
　deep inguinal lymph, 176
　inguinal lymph, 56
　ischiatic lymph, 166, 170
　mandibular lymph, 12
　prescapular lymph, 84
　superficial cervical lymph, 84
　superficial inguinal lymph, 58
Notch, acetabular, 144, 186
　greater sciatic, 140, 142
　lesser sciatic, 140, 142

Olecranon, 86
　ulnar, 112
Orifice, preputial, 56
Origin(s), of pelvic muscles, 144
Os coxae, 48, 64, 144, 202
Os pedis, 202
Ovary, 60
Oviduct, 60

Palate, hard, 14
　soft, 14
Penis, 54, 58, 174
Pericardium, 44
Perineum, 168
Periople, of hoof, 134
Peritoneum, 40, 50
Pharynx, 14
Plexus, brachial, 44, 106
　coronary venus, 116
　lumbosacral, 164, 165, 172
　pelvic, 172
　sacral, 168
Pouch, gutteral, 14
　volar, of fetlock joint, 134
Prepuce, 56
Process, articular, of 1st sacral vertebra, 140, 142
　coracoid, 68, 112
　　of scapula, 94
　　of mandible, 6
　extensor, of 3rd phalanx, 82
　medial, of fibular tarsal, 150
　olecranon, of ulna, 82, 94
　supraorbital, of frontal bone, 6
　transverse, 82
Pulse, 12, 118

Ramus communicans, 44
   mandibular, 12
Rectum, 50, 54, 60, 174
Rete carpi dorsale, 104
Rete carpi volare, 114
Ribs, 22, 36
Ring, abdominal inguinal, 54
   external inguinal, 30, 38, 40
   left subcutaneous inguinal, 56
   subcutaneous inguinal, 58
   vaginal, 50

Sacrum, 22
Scapula, 90
Scrotum, 56
Shaft, of ilium, 140, 142
Sheath, carpal, 126
   digital, 126
   digital synovial, 132, 134
   tendon, of common digital extensor, 126
      of extensor carpi obliquus, 126
      of extensor carpi radialis, 126
      of flexor carpi radialis, 126
      of lateral digital extensor, 126
Shoulder, 24, 28, 64, 108
Sinus, frontal, 8, 14
   maxillary, 8
   skeleton, 22
   sphenopalatine, 14
Skin, ventral thoracic wall, 106
Sole, of hoof, 134
Sphincter, external anal, 56, 60
Spine, scapular, 68, 82, 86
   sciatic, 140, 142
   See also Vertebrae.
Stallion, pelvic girdle, 140, 141
Sternum, 22, 30, 36, 90
Surface(s), articular, radial, 72
   ulnar, 72
Sustentaculum tali, 152
Sustentacum tali, 150
Symphysis, pelvis, 64, 140, 142, 176

Tail, 165, 168, 174
Teeth, incisor, 6, 14
   molar, 6
   premolar, 6
Tendon, of biceps brachii muscle, 102, 112, 136
   of common digital extensor muscle, 124, 134, 136
   conjoined, of latissimus dorsi and teres major muscle, 70
   of coracobrachialis muscle, 112
   cunean, 194, 200
   deep digital flexor, 128, 130
   deep flexor, 96
   of extensor carpi obliquus muscle, 94, 116, 124
   of extensor carpi radialis muscle, 112, 114, 124, 136
   of flexor carpi radialis muscle, 114, 118
   flexor carpi ulnaris, 118
   gluteus accessorius, 170
   of gluteus medius muscle, 170
   of iliopsoas muscle, 186, 188
   of lateral digital extensor muscle, 124, 196, 200
   of long digital extensor muscle, 158, 196, 198, 200
   of medial interosseous muscle, 122

Tendon—(*Cont.*)
   of obturator internus muscle, 170
   of peroneus tertius muscle, 158
   prepubic, 38, 172, 176, 182, 186
   of superficial digital flexor muscle, 116, 118, 128, 130, 134, 136
   of teres major muscle, 102
   of tibialis cranialis muscle, 198, 200
Testicle, left, 58
   right, 54
Thigh, 176
Thorax, 22
   left, 46
   right, 44
Tongue, rostral tip, 14
Trachea, 32, 34, 46
   lumen, 14
Trochanter, great, 164
   major, 146, 162
   minor, 146, 176, 182
   tertius, 146, 164, 166
Trochlea, femoral, 154
   of tibial tarsal, 200
Trunk, bicarotid, 44, 46
   sympathetic, 44, 46
Tube, Eustachian, 14
   stomach, 14
Tuber calcis, 150, 162, 178, 190, 192
Tuber coxae, 38, 40, 140, 142, 162
Tuber ischii, 142, 162, 165, 178
Tuber sacrale, 140, 142
Tuber scapulae, 102, 112
Tubercle, pubic, 140
Tuberosity, deltoid, of humerus, 70, 82, 86, 88, 92, 102, 104
   lateral, of humerus, 102, 104, 110
      of radius, 82, 104
   medial, of humerus, 90, 94, 102, 110
   metacarpal, 82, 124
   radial, 98
   scapular, 68, 98
   teres, 70
      of humerus, 90, 94
   tibial, 158
Tunic, abdominal, 90
Tunica vaginalis, 40, 58
Tunica vaginalis communis, 56

Umbilicus, 50
Ureter, 50, 60
Urethra, 54, 60
Uterus, 60

Vein(s), accessory cephalic, 92, 100, 112, 114
   angular, 10
   axillary, 44, 92, 100, 106
   azygos, 44
   brachial, 100, 109, 114
   caudal auricular, 10
   caudal circumflex humeral, 100
   caudal femoral, 166, 204
   caudal gluteal, 166
   caudal tibial, 204
   cephalic, 44, 92, 100, 112, 114, 116, 118
   circumflex scapular, 100

Vein(s)—(Cont.)
  collateral ulnar, 100, 112, 114
  costocervical, 44
  cranial circumflex humeral, 100
  cranial tibial, 204
  deep brachial, 100
  deep plantar metatarsal, 204
  deep volar metacarpal, 100
  external maxillary, 10, 12, 44
  external pudendal, 58
  external thoracic, 44, 110
  facial, 10
  femoral, 204
  intercostal, 44
  internal maxillary, 44
  internal thoracic, 44
  jugular, 4, 44, 90, 92, 100, 106
  lateral nasal, 10
  lateral superficial plantar metatarsal, 204
  lateral volar metacarpal, 100, 118
  left axillary, 46
  left jugular, 46
  masseteric, 10
  medial cubital, 100, 108, 110, 114
  medial dorsal metatarsal, 204
  medial saphenous, 204
  medial superficial plantar metatarsal, 204
  medial proper digital, 116
  medial volar metacarpal, 92, 100, 118
  median, 100, 110, 114, 116
  middle dorsal metatarsal, 204
  obturator, 116
  popliteal, 204
  precaval, 46

Vein(s)—(Cont.)
  pudendal, 166
  recurrent tarsal, 204
  recurrent tibial, 190, 204
  of rete carpi volare, 118
  saphenous, 176
  segmental intercostal, 44
  subscapular, 100, 102, 108
  superficial temporal, 10
  superior labial, 10
  suprascapular, 100
  thoracodorsal, 100, 110
  transverse facial, 10
  ulnar, 116
  vertebral, 44
Vena cava, caudal, 44, 50
  cranial, 44
Vertebra(e), atlas (1st cervical), 6
  axis (2nd cervical), 6, 22
  coccygeal, 22, 174, 178
  5th sacral, 142
  4th cervical, 82
  lumbar, 50, 172, 176
  sacral, 22
  thoracic, 22, 176
Vesicle, seminal, 54

Wall, abdominal, 32
  of hoof, 134
Wind puff(s), of fore limb, 132
Wing, of ilium, 164
  sacral, 140, 142
Withers, 22